living with a long-term illness

the facts

also available in the series

living with a long-term illness

the facts

FRANKIE CAMPLING
A person with a long-term illness

MICHAEL SHARPE
Professor of Psychological Medicine and
Symptom Research, University of
Edinburgh, Scotland, UK

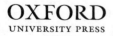

OXFORD
UNIVERSITY PRESS

OXFORD
UNIVERSITY PRESS

Great Clarendon Street, Oxford OX2 6DP

Oxford University Press is a department of the University of Oxford.
It furthers the University's objective of excellence in research, scholarship,
and education by publishing worldwide in

Oxford New York

Auckland Cape Town Dar es Salaam Hong Kong Karachi
Kuala Lumpur Madrid Melbourne Mexico City Nairobi
New Delhi Shanghai Taipei Toronto

With offices in

Argentina Austria Brazil Chile Czech Republic France Greece
Guatemala Hungary Italy Japan Poland Portugal Singapore
South Korea Switzerland Thailand Turkey Ukraine Vietnam

Oxford is a registered trade mark of Oxford University Press
in the UK and in certain other countries

Published in the United States
by Oxford University Press Inc., New York

British Library Cataloguing in Publication Data

Data available

Library of Congress Cataloging in Publication Data

Campling, Frankie.
   Living with a long-term illness : the facts / Frankie Campling, Michael Sharpe.
      p. cm.
   1. Chronic diseases—Treatment.   2. Chronically ill—Rehabilitation.
3. Self-care, Health.   I. Sharpe, Michael, 1941– .   II. Title.
RC108.C36 2006
616'.044—dc22

                                                  2005023507

Typeset by Newgen Imaging Systems (P) Ltd., Chennai, India
Printed in Great Britain
on acid-free paper by
CPI Antony Rowe, Chippenham

'N 978–0–19–852882–1 (Pbk.)

    7 6 5 4 3 2

acknowledgements

We are very grateful to those people, clinicians, health professionals and patients, who read the manuscript or who discussed the project with us, and gave us such valuable comments and suggestions. These include Lois Bennett, Hilary Briars, Diane Cox—reader in occupational medicine, Joanna Howard, Tim Jack—director of pain relief unit, Kurt Kroenke—professor of medicine, Michael von Korff—health services researcher, Roisin McClosky—general practitioner, Vanessa Strong—research nurse and David Weller—professor of general practice, though many others have given us really helpful assistance.

Most of all though, we want to thank all the people with a long-term illness with whom we have worked over the last 15 or more years. They have taught us so much about what it is like to suffer from such an illness, their problems, and what they have found helpful. This book is dedicated to them.

contents

section 3
Managing emotional issues

section 4
Managing interpersonal problems

section 5
Managing practical problems

Appendix 1

Appendix 2

Appendix 3

Index

introduction

This book is written for those people who live with a long-term illness, as well as for their carers, family and friends. We hope that the advice and information we give will be of use to them. We also hope that it will be read by doctors and other health workers and be of use to them too.

The starting point of this book is that, whatever the diagnosis, all long-term illnesses have much in common. The practical, social, and emotional problems and difficulties that are part and parcel of living with a long-term illness, and the strategies used to overcome them are shared by all sufferers.

Of course, long-term illnesses are not all exactly the same. Doctors usually categorize them by their medical diagnosis, for example diabetes, arthritis or heart disease. Patients suffering an illness, or their carers, may also usefully categorize long-term illnesses by the type of challenges they present (whether they are stable, fluctuating or possibly deteriorating), by their effect on functioning (disabling or not disabling) or by how it makes them feel (fatiguing or painful).

Our aim in writing this book is to identify the challenges posed to patients and carers by these different types of illness and to suggest a variety of ways in which you might best meet these. In order to do this, we would like you to consider becoming an expert on your illness. The concept of the 'expert (or empowered) patient'—an equal partner with his or her doctor—is one that is expanded later in the book.

We hope that this book will help you to build up your own expertise and to explore the most effective ways of helping yourself or the person you care for. Managing an illness effectively and tackling the problems and difficulties it causes can improve how you feel, what you can do and even your life experience.

Similar long-term illnesses may affect individuals differently. You are the only person who really knows how you experience it—you are already the world's greatest expert on that. We are certainly not going to say 'you **must** do such-and-such'; we respect your individual expertise and your right to make your own choices about how you manage your condition. Instead, we aim to suggest a wide variety of ideas and leave you to choose those that suit you best.

You could think of your illness as a journey and this book as a tool box, or a selection of equipment, which you can carry with you on that journey. The start of this journey was when you first noticed symptoms or got a diagnosis, and it then covers all sorts of terrain and encounters all sorts of difficulties during its course. You will need different items of equipment to help you at different stages of this journey. We hope that you will read this book with an open mind, not rejecting any of the ideas until you have given them some thought.

This book is not enough to provide all the equipment you need. We have therefore suggested many other sources of additional information, including books, websites, and audio tapes and CDs, which expand on the various topics we discuss. (You will find brief details of these at the end of chapters, but full details of them and some others are in the Further information list, Appendix 2, at the end of the book.) We have also included a small number of more scholarly references for those who are interested.

Those of our readers who have already read our previous book 'Chronic fatigue syndrome (CFS/ME): the facts' may recognize some of the themes from it in this book. This is because CFS/ME is an example of a long-term illness which has much in common with other illnesses.

You may wonder what experience and knowledge we have that gives us the right to offer advice to you. Well, this book is written by two people, one with a long-term illness and one a doctor, both of whom have had experience of being a carer. By writing this book together, we hope that we have been able to give a better all-round picture of illness than if it was written by either one of us on our own.

Though most of the writing was done jointly, there are also small pieces written just by Frankie, in which she draws on personal experience of having a long-term illness or of being a carer.

We are both British and are consequently most familiar with the medical system and social services currently existing in the UK, but we have tried to ensure that this book will be useful to readers from other countries. Internet resources in particular are international, so the websites we recommend are available to everyone.

If you would like to know the personal details of the authors of books you choose to read, we have each added short accounts of our experience of illness.

Frankie Campling—I too have a long-term illness. Until 1989 I was a busy career woman and working mother. Then I had major surgery, which was followed by chronic fatigue syndrome (CFS/ME). I had to give up my job, deal with that loss and start learning about managing an illness for which there is no medical treatment. I had been doing some telephone counselling before I became ill and this seemed to be a way in which I could continue to make a contribution in spite of my illness. At first, my callers were people like myself with CFS/ME. Later, people with other long-term conditions began to contact me, and I realized how many problems we shared.

I went on like that for some years, learning more about self-management. I started writing about CFS/ME and about illness in general. Some of the time, I preach rather better than I practice. I cannot say that I always manage myself as well as I could, but perhaps that gives me some insight into how other people can get pushed away from what is the best way of managing their own condition.

In 1997, things changed. My husband became ill with a heart condition that required a by-pass operation. He had had an arthritic knee for many years, which became increasingly painful and disabling. I had to make the transition from being the one cared for to being the carer. Finally, he was diagnosed as having cancer and, in spite of having chemotherapy and major surgery, he died in 2002. This was not my only experience of being a carer; before I became ill, my father-in-law, suffering from Alzheimer's disease, lived with us for a year. I remember very vividly just how difficult that was.

I met Michael Sharpe in 1990 when he was doing research into CFS/ME in Oxford. He helped me with the patient information booklet I wrote on CFS/ME and we later collaborated on a book on the subject. I think we make a good team.

Michael Sharpe—I am a doctor and a medical researcher with wide experience of chronic illness. I did my first degree in Psychology and then spent a period in laboratory research before training in Medicine. Although I very much enjoyed my training in general medicine, I became increasingly frustrated by the emphasis on the biology of disease and the failure of the medical system to address chronic illness from the patient's perspective. I therefore chose to train in psychiatry in order to supplement my general medical knowledge. I have gone on to develop a particular interest in research into the management of chronic conditions.

This research has included studies of the experience and treatment of people following stroke, as well as those with cancer, chronic fatigue syndrome and other conditions. I am currently working with neurologists, cancer specialists and primary care doctors in an effort to develop better treatments, especially self-help treatments, for chronic illnesses and the symptoms they present. I have come to understand that dividing illness into either a physical or a psychological type is unhelpful, and that all illness, particularly chronic illness, is affected by both physical and psychological factors. My aim is to achieve more genuinely integrated (biopsychosocial) medical care for patients with chronic conditions, and to encourage a type of medicine which takes full account of the patient's own subjective experience and what they can do, as well as the biology of their disease and how that can be treated.

I am Professor of Psychological Medicine and Symptoms Research in the University of Edinburgh and Fellow of the Royal College of Physicians of London, the Royal College of Physicians of Edinburgh, the Royal College of Psychiatrists of the UK and the Academy of Psychosomatic Medicine (USA). I am married with two children, and have also had my fair share of chronic illness in members of my family. As a teenager, I nursed my grandfather in his terminal illness. I have subsequently witnessed the nature, challenges and effects of chronic illness and death in a number of close relatives and friends, and have been deeply touched by how these people have risen to the challenges, each in their own way.

I have written several academic books, but found that writing the first book with Frankie Campling—'Chronic fatigue syndrome (CFS/ME): the facts'— produced something that I do not think either of us could have written alone. I was therefore most keen to work with her again on this book, in which we address the much broader challenge of long-term illness in general.

section 1
Long-term illness and you

1 What is long-term (chronic) illness?

As its title suggests, this book is about long-term (chronic) illness, as opposed to short-term (acute) illness, and about how a long-term illness can best be managed. Before we move on to talk about illness management though, we would like to start by discussing a few other topics which we believe will help you understand the approach we are taking.

Illness and how it differs from disease

You may have noticed that in the Introduction, we used the word 'illness' rather than 'disease'. Disease is actually not the same as illness. This distinction between disease and illness is fundamental to our approach for helping you manage your own illness. So what is the difference?

- Disease refers to the changes in your body that the doctor identifies (on examination or with medical tests). It is *the doctor's* objective findings of changes that are common to all people with a particular disease and which are described in medical textbooks.

- Illness refers to your experience of being unwell. It describes your symptoms, your reactions to them, and what you can or cannot do. It is *your own* personal subjective experience. In other words, there is much more to illness than just disease.

You might think that disease and illness always go together. Surprisingly, they do not. For example, it is quite possible to have a disease (such as cancer) without feeling ill at all, and many people feel ill even though doctors can find no disease. What is more, people with the very same disease typically suffer very different degrees of illness.

You may feel that all this is just splitting hairs. You personally may not care whether what you suffer from is called a disease or an illness. However, making this distinction opens up a new perspective on your ill health and offers new ways for you to help yourself.

The integrated or biopsychosocial approach to illness

It is useful if you (and your doctors) can think about your illness in the broadest possible way, looking at all the things that contribute to how unwell you feel. If you only think about the disease process that may be associated with your particular illness, you limit the way in which you can help yourself or be helped. It is useful to consider a variety of other aspects of the illness.

One such integrated view of illness has been called the biopsychosocial approach, which sounds like something very scientific and complicated. Actually it is quite a common-sense approach. It takes into account all the things (sometimes called 'factors') that can cause a person to feel unwell, and groups them for convenience sake into *bio*logical, *psycho*logical and *social* categories. This can be very much to the point in understanding and managing a long-term illness. By considering *all* the relevant 'factors', and not just the changes in your body that could enable a doctor to diagnose a disease, it helps you to understand what else may be causing your feeling of illness, as well as all the things that you and your doctor can do to make you feel better. (Remember how we defined 'illness'—your *own* experience of being unwell.)

How can things from these three categories have an effect on the way that you feel?

- *Biological*—the biological (or physical) factors that cause you to feel unwell can include an identified disease, i.e. something faulty in some part of your body. For example, in diabetes, the pancreas does not make enough insulin and, in cancer, there is an uncontrolled growth of cells. However, there can be other physical factors that contribute to how a person with a long-term illness feels. These include changes in how well your body works (or functions). For example, if you become very inactive, this can mean that your muscles, heart and lungs function less efficiently, leading you to experience a loss of 'physical fitness'.

- *Psychological*—all long-term illnesses affect how people think, how they feel emotionally and how they behave, which can then have an effect on their feelings of being unwell. Psychological factors include your thinking, your emotions and what behaviours you use to cope with your illness. For example, if you worry about or focus too much on your symptoms (such as pain), they will probably feel more severe. If you become depressed or anxious, this alters the way your brain works and also makes symptoms feel worse. How you cope plays an especially important part. For example, if you avoid all activities, you could become demoralized or even depressed. If you are coping well, you will probably feel better too.

- *Social and interpersonal*—nobody exists in isolation. The way that we interact with other people and how they respond to us will influence what help we get and how we feel. What others say or do, and how much support we get influences how we feel psychologically. Wider social factors such as generally accepted views about certain illnesses can make the illness experience feel worse.

The fact that many things other than disease can make you feel unwell sounds bad. In fact, it is actually a good thing. It means that, even if you have no identified disease or if your disease cannot be cured, there are still a great many other areas that you can work on to improve the way that you feel. The bottom line is that as well as getting the best possible medical treatment for your *disease* (if one can be found), there is a whole range of things you can do to improve your *illness*.

This biopsychosocial approach helps to identify all the things that could make you feel ill, but it also suggests how these things affect each other— how they interact. For example, if you become worried about your health, you may stop going out and become less active. Being less active may lead to you becoming more isolated and depressed. All of these things can have an effect on how well your body functions.

BIOLOGICAL FACTORS
(disease and other bodily changes)

ILLNESS

PSYCHOLOGICAL
FACTORS
(thoughts, mood and coping)

SOCIAL & INTERPERSONAL
FACTORS
(support and attitudes to illness)

Figure 1.1 Factors that shape illness

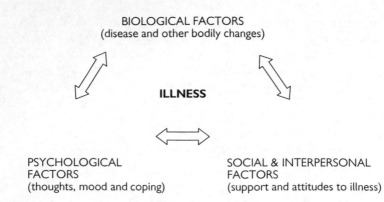

Figure 1.2 Interactions of factors that shape illness

Understanding that these factors interact with each other is helpful. It means that you do not need to work on all the things causing your illness; working on one or two can change the others. For example, a positive attitude to coping with the illness may enable you to be more active, improve what you can do and how you feel, and make your body work better.

Remember that people are very different. For a given person, some factors are more important than others. They do not all apply to everyone. The aim of this book is to help you understand what is important in *your* illness. You might find it helpful to start to think about what factors are relevant to your illness. When you know that, you will be in a much better position to start thinking about how to manage your package in the best way.

2 Long-term illness as a journey

Long-term illness can be thought of as a journey, which started when you first noticed symptoms or when you were given a diagnosis. Diagnosis can be such an important part of your journey that it is worth looking more closely at what it might mean to you.

Diagnosis

A diagnosis can be important if it helps you to understand why you have been feeling the way you have. It may be the end of a search to discover what is causing the symptoms you have noticed, perhaps for some time. It may be a confirmation of something you have suspected, or it can come as a complete surprise.

If the diagnosis is of a long-term illness, it is not just an end point. It is also the beginning of a long journey. The need to embark on such a journey is rarely welcome. Indeed, it usually comes as an unpleasant shock. If you have believed that other people get ill but not you, or that doctors can always cure illness, you may feel anger and disappointment when this turns out not to be true in your case. If the diagnosis is of something potentially life threatening, then fear of death is added to your reaction. Even if you were fairly certain about what would be diagnosed, having your suspicions finally confirmed can still be alarming. No two people, even if they have the same illness, experience diagnosis in exactly the same way. Your particular experience is unique.

Once a diagnosis is made, it often takes time for the full message to sink in. It may take a while for you to realize fully how much things may change—that there is no going back to before you got the diagnosis. For some people, the process can be traumatic; for others, it is easier. If you are reading this book, it is likely that you have already been through this process. You, as the world's greatest expert on you, will know what it was like, how you coped and what would have made things easier. We hope that you got all the support you needed. It is worth remembering what it was like. It is the nature of life that you may get further diagnoses—a new stage in your particular illness or something else to add to it. Remembering how you reacted earlier may help you cope better next time. Perhaps you would do the same again, but perhaps you would need a different approach, maybe being more gentle and kind to yourself. Perhaps you could be more explicit with others about your need for support.

Mary had been getting pain in her hips for some time and was fairly certain that it was caused by osteoarthritis. Nevertheless, she found that getting the official diagnosis left her feeling upset and miserable. She was rather stern with herself, saying things like 'For goodness sake stop being so feeble. You knew beforehand what they were going to tell you. There's no reason to be miserable.' Years later, after she had had two hip replacements, she developed osteoarthritis in her shoulders. This time she was kinder to herself and accepted that it was perfectly normal to feel depressed about getting that diagnosis. She was careful to do all that she could to cherish herself and was more definite about asking for support.

An alarming diagnosis

Certain diagnoses can be particularly alarming. Some of you reading this may already have received an alarming diagnosis—perhaps something like cancer or another illness with a frightening prognosis. You may have found that your ideas about yourself and your future suddenly became very different. You may well have felt shocked or numb, or found it hard to accept what you had been told. Some people feel very angry about the apparent unfairness of it and find themselves questioning 'Why me? What have I ever done to deserve this?' Different people cope with these emotions in different ways, but it is important to believe that no way is the wrong way.

Even if you have been given an alarming diagnosis like cancer and received successful treatment, the effects of having had such a disease can be long term. Most people continue to fear that the cancer could return and so *any* new symptom can feel alarming. The treatment may have caused long-term symptoms such as fatigue or changes in your body. Such symptoms or changes need to be managed positively. You will find more about this later in the book.

One emotional effect of an alarming diagnosis is getting stuck in fear or anger. There are ways to deal with this. It may ease your feelings if you can talk about this to someone with whom you feel comfortable. Writing down your feelings may help too. You may be able to get specialized counselling to help you deal with the problem, perhaps through your hospital clinic. Some people who have got stuck in thinking 'why me?' have found it helpful to consider the opposite question 'why not me?' You certainly do not have to feel that something in your past makes you deserve illness, and you have every right to resent anyone suggesting such a thing.

Another way in which some people deal with an alarming diagnosis is to shut their minds to it, to deny it. Denial may be an appropriate response for you, at least for a time, as long as it does not stop you managing the symptoms of your illness or getting the necessary treatment.

A non-disease diagnosis

There are, unfortunately, many illnesses which are not caused by any known disease (they do not produce changes in the body that can be identified on available tests). Chronic fatigue and chronic pain syndromes are well known examples. Knowing that you are ill but not having a definite label for what is wrong can make life especially difficult. It can be hard to cope with something if you do not know what it is. However, you may have to accept that, with the limitations of medical science, you may never have a simple disease diagnosis.

Some doctors (and other people) tend to think that if a disease cannot be identified, then you are not really ill. They may even say that it is 'all in your mind', not a real illness and blame you for it. This is simply a failure on their part to distinguish between disease and illness. After reading this book, you may be able to explain this to them—you may not have a *disease* that can be diagnosed, but you do have a real *illness*. If you, your family, your friends and your doctor are able to accept that you really are ill, even if it is not possible to identify changes in your body with medical tests, then together you can start the process of working out how to manage the illness.

Of course you would prefer to have a clear-cut disease diagnosis. If nothing else, it would make it easier to explain your illness to those around you—family, friends or employers—or to get benefits. Whilst it is possible that, in time, new tests might be developed or your symptoms might change in a way that makes it easier to identify what is wrong with your body, this is often not the case. Some people spend a great deal of energy, not to mention money, in a continuing search for the doctor who will find out what is wrong and offer a cure. All too frequently, this is a vain hope that gets in the way of getting on with actively managing your illness. If you can accept the uncertainty and settle down to *managing* your illness in spite of the lack of a label, you may well be surprised by how much you can improve it.

The journey

You may find it helpful to explore this idea a little more. The journey is probably not one which you intended to make; it diverted you away from quite another journey—the one you expected to make as a well person. There will probably be times when you bitterly resent having to travel along your new path and long to return to the one you hoped or expected to be making. Unfortunately, you simply do not have that choice, so the question becomes one of how can you make the best of the journey you are actually on.

It can sometimes help to think in terms of a real journey into unknown territory. If you were starting off on such a journey, how would you prepare for it, what equipment and assistance would you want? Here are some ideas to get you started. You might want:

A map—some idea of the final destination and the route towards it

An informed guide—someone who has knowledge of the territory and the best routes across it

Companions on the journey—people alongside you on your travels

Appropriate travel equipment—such as the right clothes and shoes for the terrain you were crossing

Supplies—food and housing along the way

Rest houses—places and times to pause and rest.

This way of thinking can help you identify what help and support would make things easier for you. You may not get all that you want or need, but at least you would have a better idea of what you could ask for. These things could include information, help, treatment, coaching, equipment, companionship, love, and inspiration.

One thing that some people have found helpful is actually to draw a map or chart of their journey through illness so far. There are different ways of doing this, but one simple way is to draw a line down a page and then put against it the moments that were significant to you, whether good or bad. This can help you get a clearer picture of where you have been and, perhaps, where you are going. You might be able to add something to your map about where you think you will go next.

It could be done in a purely medical way—'I first noticed symptoms in year X. I got a diagnosis in year Y', etc. However, you could also add things that had personal significance that were not directly associated with your illness—'my daughter got married in year Z'. You might put in times when you overcame obstacles, or moments of loss or triumph. This is *your* map, so you could do it in any way that works for you. You may well find that, once you have done a first draft, it gets you thinking about other significant events or emotions that you could add.

Here are two examples:

James' map of his journey through heart problems

1997 I started experiencing chest pains after exertion. My doctor diagnosed angina, and prescribed a drug to use when I got the pain.

1998 The pain began to occur more frequently and to be more severe. My doctor referred me to a heart specialist at our local hospital.

1998 I was seen by the specialist, who put me on the waiting list to have an angiogram, followed if necessary by an angioplasty.

1999 The angiogram showed that I had blocked veins in my heart, but the angioplasty was not successful. I was put on the waiting list for a heart by-pass operation.

2000 I had a triple by-pass operation. This was very successful, but I still have other medical problems—type 2 diabetes and an arthritic knee. My doctor and I will have to go on managing them.

Mary's map of her journey through osteoarthritis

1987 Started noticing pain in my hips

1988 Pain increasing. Using painkillers regularly. Suspected that it was osteoarthritis. Pain is very tiring. It is getting in the way of my work as a management trainer. Saw myself on a class video and was horrified at how disabled I looked hobbling round.

1990 Diagnosis of osteoarthritis confirmed, which was surprisingly upsetting as I'd suspected that. Told myself I was being silly. Saw surgeon who agreed to do hip replacements, even though I was young for it, to allow me to go on working and earning my living.

1990 Right hip replaced. Though the operation was successful, the six weeks after when I couldn't drive made working very difficult. I don't like having to ask for help.

1991 Left hip replaced. Freedom from pain was wonderful. Felt like a new woman, or rather the woman I used to be. Was better this time about asking for help after the operation.

1996 Shoulders beginning to be painful. Diagnosis of osteoarthritis there was again surprisingly depressing. Found myself a good counsellor with whom I could discuss this. Stiffness in my shoulders made it hard t dress myself and so I found problems in finding smart working clot' that I could get on.

1997 Began to have problems with taking NSAIDs, which upset my stomach. With my doctor's help found other painkillers that worked almost as well.

2001 Signs that right replacement hip joint needs revising.

2002 Right hip joint very painful. Needing to use a crutch all the time. Now clients are beginning to say 'poor you' which I hate. The body bit isn't important. My brain is just as good as ever.

2003 Operation to revise right hip fairly successful, but I still need to use a crutch some of the time. I mind this less now. Being able to get about and to work is what is important.

2004 Concentrating more on work that I can do at home and on the computer, so as to have less need to travel. Started writing a novel, quite a change from the academic books I've written before. This might be something I could develop in the future.

3 Gathering information and becoming an 'expert patient'

What is an 'expert patient'?

'Expert patients' are people suffering with a long-term illness who have chosen to become well informed about how to manage both their disease and their illness. They may do this in two ways—firstly by finding out as much as possible about its causes, management, and prognosis, and by experimenting to see what suits them; secondly, they may work towards managing their illness in a partnership with their doctors. Another way of describing 'expert patients' is to call them 'empowered patients'. They have chosen to take as much control over their illness and their lives as is possible and appropriate.

We do want to stress that you have a choice. Not everybody wants to know all the technical details of their disease. Some people feel more comfortable leaving this to their doctors and just knowing what those doctors have chosen to tell them. If this is the way that you feel, then that is a choice you are entitled to make. Though you may choose not to become an expert on the medical details of your own disease, we do recommend that you become an expert on the management of your illness. That is really what this book is about.

Inevitably, every patient becomes an expert in one aspect of their illness—how it affects them. Nobody can know this better than you!

If you have one of the less common long-term illnesses, you may have come to know more about it than your family doctors, though that does not mean that they do not have a lot to offer you. Even without knowing as much as you about that particular illness, they can help you with symptom management and with evaluating information you have found for yourself. In Chapter 27, we talk about the best ways of sharing some of your knowledge with your doctor.

Sources of information

There is no one complete source of information. You may need to access a variety of sources to get the complete picture—like assembling pieces of a mosaic. Some of the sources could be:

- Your family doctor and the health team in the practice. You can ask them for information and they may have useful leaflets to offer.

- A hospital clinic, if you attend one. Your specialist and the clinic nurses will be able to give you information about your particular illness, and may well have information booklets, books or videos available.

- Other health professionals such as health visitors, physiotherapists and occupational therapists.

- The national support group for your illness. This can often be a valuable source of information.

- Books about your particular illness. Be wary though. Some of these will reflect individual sufferers' experience of the illness which may or may not be relevant to your own experience.

- Other people with the same illness. You may meet them because you both attend the same clinic, or through a local support group. Again, remember that they will often speak from their own experiences, which may be different from yours.

- Things you read or hear from the media—magazine or newspaper articles, radio or TV programmes. However, as with support groups, journalists do tend to concentrate on extremes.

- Telephone help lines, run either by a national support group or by organizations such as NHS Direct.

- Disability organizations.

- And, finally, the Internet, which is so important that it deserves a section of its own—so it gets one here.

The Internet as a source of information

More and more people are turning to the Internet as a source of information about many things, including their illness. It is not necessary to own a computer to do this—many public libraries have computer facilities that can be used by the public, and there are Internet cafes in most high streets where you can 'surf the net' for a modest fee.

Although the following box (Box 3.1) concerns cancer patients' use of the Internet, many of the reasons given in it can be applied to other illnesses.

Box 3.1 When and why cancer patients use the Internet

Before visiting their doctor—To discover the possible meaning of symptoms

During investigations—To seek reassurance that the doctor is doing the right test, to prepare for results, to improve the value of the consultation, to avoid esprit d'escalier*

After the diagnosis—To gather information about the cancer (including information that is 'difficult' to ask about directly), to seek advice about how to tell children, to contact online support groups, to seek second opinions, to make sense of the stages of the disease, to interpret what professionals have said, to tackle isolation

When choosing treatments—Information about treatment options and side effects, experimental treatments, research, and alternative and complementary treatments

Before treatment—To find out what to take to hospital, what will happen, and what it will be like, what to expect of recovery, how to identify and to prepare questions to ask the doctors

Short-term follow up—Information about side effects, reassurance about symptoms, advice about diet, complementary treatment, advice on benefits and finances, to check that the treatment was optimal, perceived therapeutic benefits

Long-term follow up—To share experience and advice, contact support groups and chat rooms, to campaign about the condition, to make anonymous inquiries.

(*'an apt or clever remark that comes to mind after the chance to make it has gone') *Concise Oxford Dictionary*

From the article 'How the internet affects patients' experience of cancer: a qualitative study, Ziebland *et al.*, 2004, reproduced by permission of the *British Medical Journal*.

You can search for information on your illness by looking for websites dealing with that subject. Another way is to go to the general medical information websites and then look in them for your illness. The advantage of doing it that way is that you can know that the information has been carefully vetted and is reliable. There are some websites of this type that we can recommend:

- www.nhsdirect.nhs.uk
- www.ebandolier.org.uk
- www.mayoclinic.com

- www.healthtalk.com
- www.medic8.com

You can find information about drugs by looking at:

- www.bnf.org. This is the website of the *British National Formulary* (a book of medicines used in the UK). You may have seen the book on your doctor's desk.
- www.intelihealth.com. This is the website for the *US Pharmacopoeia* (an American book of medicines).

The national patient support organizations for individual illnesses mostly have their own websites. These can often be a good source of information.

Another source of information and support on the Internet is the discussion lists (support groups) and chat rooms for different illnesses and diseases. Here, patients exchange information and support each other. Some people find them extremely useful. Once you have signed up for the list, copies of all messages are sent to your e-mail address. You may find the volume of mail a bit overwhelming, but with experience you will soon find ways of picking out the bits that interest you.

Further information

The Patient's Internet Handbook, by Robert Killey and Elizabeth Graham, gives really helpful information on how to search the web for information and how to evaluate information you find. It has a list of the 100 most common illnesses with details of support groups, online discussion groups and other helpful information. You can find details of this book in Appendix 2.

Evaluating the information you find

It is easy enough to gather a mass of information about your illness. What is not so easy is to assess just how accurate it is and how relevant it is to you. Some of it will be good quality and really pertinent to you and your illness, but some can be frankly misleading. How are you to judge?

One 'tool' that will help you judge and which we can thoroughly recommend is the DISCERN Instrument www.discern.org.uk/discern_ intrument. This is a series of 15 questions that you should ask yourself as you read through anything about treatment choices. We have been allowed ⇒ reproduce it in this book, and you will find the whole thing in ⸱ᵖendix 1. Each question is accompanied by tips and hints to help you answer it. Though it was originally created to help patients deal with printed information, it can be applied just as much to what you read on the Internet. Do have a look at it. If you can look at the website as well, you will find that it gives more advice on how to answer each question.

Research into treatments (clinical trials)

You may well read about new treatments for your disease or illness. One of the factors you would need to weigh up would be the quality of any research that has been carried out on such treatments.

Clinical trials

You may read about a treatment for your illness, and notice that it says 'medical trials have shown'. How much weight you give to this depends on what kind of trials they were. It is worth knowing a bit more about trials. Before a treatment can be recommended as being of proved effectiveness, it must have been properly tested. The 'gold standard' of such tests is a randomized, controlled trial (RCT). High quality evidence from RCTs should include the following:

- Trials with a random allocation of patients (i.e. by chance, as by tossing a coin) to one of two treatment groups; one group being given the new treatment and the other another treatment (sometimes a placebo, sometimes the usual care). This makes certain that the patients in both groups are similar.

- Trials that involve a comparison with another treatment (which is what controlled means). To see if the treatment is better, and not harmful, it must be compared with an existing treatment or no treatment.

- Trials where the patients' outcome was measured blind to which treatment the individual patients received, so that judgement of the degree of improvement is not biased by enthusiasm for the new treatment.

- Trials that were large (preferably hundreds rather than tens of patients), so that they can include a wide range of patients and minimize the possibility that any difference (or lack of difference) is due to chance.

- Trials that have been replicated. A single RCT may produce 'fluke' results, but if when it is repeated in another centre it produces the same results it is more likely to be reliable.

- Finally, the long-term effects of the treatment should be monitored to see how long the benefit lasts and to ensure that no harmful effects become apparent that were not revealed in the short-term trials.

So if you read something like '16 patients were tried with drug X and reported an improvement in their symptoms', then this might be an interesting early observation, but not something that should necessarily make you change your existing treatment. That would need better evidence.

What is a placebo?

We mentioned placebos earlier. The word placebo literally means 'I please' and is used in two different ways. One refers to an inactive pill used in trials of new drugs. In such trials, half the patients are given the drug being tested and half a placebo (the inactive pill) that looks just the same as the drug being tested. The difference in response shows whether it is the active ingredient in the drug that is making people feel better or simply the effect of being given a pill.

The placebo effect refers both to the effects of the placebo medicine (the narrow placebo effect) and to the effect of the whole procedure of medical assessment, advice, support and the giving of a prescription (the wide placebo effect).

The wide placebo effect can be strong. In trials of new drugs to relieve symptoms, it is common for as many as 30% of the patients to report a benefit (and side effects!). In research, this is a nuisance that complicates the evaluation of new drugs and makes placebo-controlled trials necessary.

In practice, it points to an important ingredient of all medical care. A good healing relationship between the doctor or therapist and the patient can in itself be helpful. It has also been noted that if the doctor or therapist and the patient believe that the treatment given is effective, it is much more likely to be so. This is probably one way that some alternative therapies which do not involve the giving of active chemicals work, especially if both the therapist and the patient have faith in the treatment. So the wider placebo effect is not something to be merely dismissed, but something that can help.

Causes for wariness

Just because something has been printed or appears on a website does not mean that it is accurate, reliable or unbiased. Do remember that anyone can start a website. There is no authority vetting all these thousands of sites, though there are some sites that have been given a rating by the Health on the Net Foundation. Some things to watch out for, whether in a printed text or on an Internet site should be:

- How recent is the information? Is there anything that would give you an indication of when the information was assembled? Something that was written some time ago may now be out of date.

- Is there any indication of where the information has come from? Are there references to recent books or to papers in reputable medical journals?

- Who is producing the web site? Do they have an axe to grind? Many do.

- Is the site trying to sell you something? If so, the information may be slanted towards making a sale.

- Is the information one sided or biased, giving you only part of the picture?

- Is the site pushing a 'miracle cure'? If you have been told by your doctors that, in the present state of medical knowledge, they cannot offer you a cure, then you should be very sceptical about cures offered on the Internet.

- Does the information come from a reputable medical source or is it one person's view of what has helped them?

If you intend to show your doctor some of the information you have gathered, then the source of the information is particularly important. A doctor is much more likely to give weight to something from a reputable source.

4 Managing disease

If your illness is associated with a disease, part of managing your illness is to manage your disease. This requires that you get the right disease diagnosis, obtain and accept treatment for it, and monitor your progress. For a long-term illness, treatment for the disease almost always involves the people who are suffering from it taking an active part. For example, in diabetes, people have to check their blood sugar themselves and use diet, insulin or medicine appropriately. How well this is done influences not only how well you feel, but also the progress of the disease itself. Managing disease on an on-going basis is an essential part, though only a part, of managing your illness.

Common long-term (chronic) diseases

There are very many long-term (chronic) diseases. Here is a list of some of the most common ones:

Diabetes mellitus
Thyroid disease
Multiple sclerosis (MS)
Functional weakness
Stroke
Heart disease
High blood pressure (hypertension)
Cancer
Chronic fatigue syndrome (CFS/ME)
Chronic pain
Chronic headache
Arthritis (osteo- and rheumatoid)
Irritable bowel syndrome
Inflammatory bowel disease
Psoriasis
Eczema

Asthma
Chronic bronchitis

This is not a complete list. We apologize if we have not included the disease from which you suffer.

Getting medical help

The help you get from your doctors is important, as well as what you do to help yourself. However, chronic (long-term) illness is very different from acute (short-term) illness and needs a different kind of management. Doctors are mainly trained to deal with acute illness, and many hospital services are organized to care for it. This means that you will often have to take an active part in getting the help that you need.

One thing that you can do to improve the relationship is to impress on your doctors that even if they cannot cure you, they can help you with managing your symptoms (for which you are grateful). That can give them a sense of effectiveness.

What help can doctors offer to a long-term patient? They can:

- Do tests
- Support you and monitor your progress
- Make referrals to other doctors or to others in the health care team
- Help you judge information about your illness that you have found for yourself
- Suggest treatment for some conditions—usually drugs
- Diagnose some other condition you may develop
- Perhaps suggest surgical treatment.

We talk more about your relationship with doctors and about the help that they can offer in Chapter 27.

Drug therapy

Drugs can be important in managing your disease, such as the use of insulin in diabetes. They can also help to control some of the symptoms of the condition, such as taking analgesic drugs for pain, or antidepressants for depression.

You may be reluctant to take drugs at all or find the side effects distressing. However, rather than deny yourself a useful source of help, you could discuss these issues with your doctor to see if a solution could be found.

There might be another drug that has fewer side effects, or taking the drug in a different way or at a different time might help. It is in your own interest not to accept a prescription and then fail to take the drug, while leaving your doctor with the impression that you are taking it.

If you are taking supplements or herbal remedies, do let your doctor know about them. Some of these could conflict with your prescribed drugs.

You could find out more about prescribed medicines or interactions between them and supplements by talking to a pharmacist, reading the *British National Formulary* or looking at one of the websites we recommend.

It can be tempting to believe that there must be *something* you could take, whether a prescription drug or a supplement, which would make things much better. Many people spend a lot of time searching the Internet for suggestions. Being open to ideas can be a good thing, but it can distract you from other ways of managing your condition that could be more helpful.

Difficulties with taking drugs

Even if you have been prescribed drugs to help in the management of your disease, you may have reservations about taking them. Simply not taking the prescribed drugs would not be the best way of managing things. 'Non-compliance/non-adherence' (a doctor's term) is a major problem across the whole spectrum of disease and illness, and is a very complex subject. Some of the reasons people do not take the medicines they have been prescribed are the following:

- *Fear or dislike of side effects*—sometimes doctors prescribe a medication without explaining just why it is important or what it is intended to achieve. That then makes it difficult to balance out the likely benefits against possible unpleasant side effects. Make sure you get enough information about why you need a medicine, even if it means asking your doctor further questions. The information leaflets that come with any drug are required to list all known side effects (which can be very frightening), but some of these will be very rare. Again, do discuss this with your doctor or with your pharmacist.

- *Dislike of taking any medicine*—some people really dislike taking any medicine. While it can be sensible to keep to as few drugs as possible, some medicines may be essential to the management of your condition. Do ask whether a particular drug could just help a bit or whether it essential in your condition. Find out what would be likely to ha if you do not take a particular drug.

- *Forgetfulness*—It can be only too easy to forget to take your drugs some of the time. It can be helpful if you can set up a routine to help you remember. There are pill boxes that you can buy which are labelled with the days of the week, so that you can check if you have taken today's pills. You could tie taking your pills in with something else that you do remember, like taking them at the same time as you clean your teeth. You could ask someone who lives with you to remind you. If you have a mobile phone, you could set up an alarm call at the appropriate time.

- *Not wanting to admit that you really do have a medical problem*—not accepting the reality of your medical condition, at least some of the time, is common in long-term illness. This is one of the negative effects of denial.

Further information

www.bnf.org. The website for the *British National Formulary*

www.intelihealth.com. The website for the *US Pharmacopoeia*

Help with diet

There are many diseases in which sticking to a certain special diet can be very important. Diabetes, coeliac disease and renal failure are just a few examples. You are likely to be given advice by your hospital clinic, or by your family doctor. You could also ask to be referred to a dietician. Talking with other people who have the same problems can often give you useful information on how to incorporate these dietary rules in your normal life.

Surgical help

You may be offered an operation as part of your medical treatment. It is worth finding out as much as you can about a particular operation before you decide to go ahead with it. It can be very tempting to think that surgery would be the complete answer to all your problems, but this is frequently not the case. For example, surgical treatment for back pain may help, but it may not. A basic question could be whether the operation is essential or whether it might just control some symptoms. Obviously, you are unlikely to refuse a life-saving operation, but you might want to weigh up the pros and cons of others. You certainly have right to ask about the chances of success, possible adverse effects and could go wrong.

As well as talking to your doctor or surgeon, you could also find out more, perhaps by talking to someone you know who has had that operation, or by talking to a helpline such as NHS Direct.

You should also feel free to discuss whether it is essential to have it right away, or whether there would be benefits in leaving it till later. An example of this could be a hip replacement, which if you are still fairly young might have to be revised in later years. Other questions you might need to ask could be what the hospital record is like for infections and what experience your surgeon has with that particular procedure.

If you do decide to go ahead with surgery, doing some forward planning is a good idea. You would need to be in the best possible shape before you go into hospital. Recovery from surgery requires a lot of energy. You may not feel much like eating in the first few days after surgery, so being underweight beforehand will not help your recovery. Make certain that you are eating really well in the weeks before the operation and once you get home. Check with your doctor or surgeon whether you need to come off some of your routine drugs or supplements in the weeks before surgery. An example could be if you are taking aspirin regularly, which could cause bleeding.

You may be offered physiotherapy to help you deal with some of the effects of the operation. Do try to cooperate with this. Getting back into the best possible physical shape will certainly help you.

Convalescence is not a fashionable concept these days. Nevertheless, it is frequently necessary and important. You need to plan for it and to accept that it may take some weeks or months before you get back to normal again. You may well take longer to recover than would someone who was fully fit to begin with. Any extra help you can get during this period is going to be especially valuable, and this may need to be planned in advance.

Further information

NHS Direct

www.besttreatments.co.uk. A website organized by the British Medical Association.

www.pocketdoctor.co.uk. This gives lists of sensible questions to ask before surgery.

Help from the health care team

There are a number of different health care specialities who may be a give you assistance in the management of your illness. Your famil is often the gatekeeper to such services, though you may be offered such help by a hospital clinic. They could include:

- Nurse specialists—many hospital clinics and doctor's surgeries have such nurses attached to them. They can be a very good source of information and advice about the problems associated with your particular illness
- Physiotherapists—they can advise you on ways to keep your body in the best shape possible, or perhaps help in some form of rehabilitation
- Occupational therapists—they can show you how to undertake specific activities that will help you reach your maximum level of functioning. They can also advise on equipment and aids around the house to make your life easier. Depending on their local budgets, they may be able to provide and install such equipment, but often their main role is to offer advice
- Dieticians—they can help if you need special diets because of your illness or if you have the problem of being under- or overweight
- Pharmacists—the pharmacist in your local chemist shop can give you information about drugs you have been prescribed and discuss any side effects
- Speech and language therapists—they can be very helpful if you have problems with your speech, for instance after a stroke, or if your condition means that you have difficulties with such things as swallowing
- Social workers—they can look at the whole picture of your illness and suggest what help might be available
- Chiropodists—taking good care of your feet might be a vital ingredient of your illness management, particularly in such illnesses as diabetes
- Opticians—having regular checks on your eyes can be very important not only in diabetes, but to catch conditions such as glaucoma
- Continence advisors—if you are having bladder or bowel problems, it is well worth seeking advice from a continence clinic, rather than trying to manage them on your own

Think about what problems and difficulties you are experiencing. If you do not feel that you are getting adequate help with them, then it could be worth talking to your doctor or specialist about being referred to one of the health professionals we have listed.

5 Managing illness

This book is essentially about *managing* your illness. Management includes both medical management and your own self-management. Active self-management of your illness is an opportunity to improve your quality of life that should not be missed.

Of course, it is tempting to expect someone else, such as your doctor or specialist, to do all of the work for you. For some acute illnesses that might even be possible, but for a long-term illness there is a lot that *only you* can do. It is a matter of taking responsibility for those parts of your illness which are under your control.

The ideal is a balance between what you can do and what your doctor can do—a collaboration between the two of you, with you as an equal partner. What cannot be cured does not have to be just endured; it can be managed—by you.

Why bother with self-management?

There are a lot of good reasons why it is worth making the effort to do what you can to help yourself.

Fewer or less severe symptoms

By managing yourself and your illness in the best way, you may well get the benefit of a reduction of some of your symptoms, particularly those such as fatigue, pain or sleep problems.

An increase in the amount you are able to do

By managing the way in which you do things or the timing of your activities, it is very probable that you will find that you can achieve rather more.

Improving your prognosis

If you have a condition that could deteriorate, then self-management could help. You might be able to avoid deterioration, reduce it or delay it. This is something well worth discussing with your doctor. Find out as much as you can about what you could do to improve your prognosis.

Feeling more in control of your life

Believing that you are not just a helpless victim is very important to your self-esteem and well-being. Knowing that you really can do something to help yourself can be a definite boost to the way you feel about yourself and your illness.

Change

You may well find that, in order to get the best out of your new life, you need to make changes; some of these changes may not be easy. It is natural to cling on to the memory of what you used to be and what you used to be able to do, and this can hold you back.

Dealing with a new stage in your illness or deciding on a self-management programme also involves change. So perhaps it could be useful to look more closely at the process of change.

In organizations, eight stages of change have been identified. Each of these stages must be gone through if the change is going to be successfully achieved. These stages apply just as much to illness and are worth looking at more closely.

- *Reluctance*—people often feel uneasy about change. They want to stay where they are, so the prospect of change is unwelcome. Certainly, having to adapt to being unwell can be very unwelcome.
- *Awareness*—coming to terms with the fact that change is simply inevitable, however much you resent it. Developing a full awareness of your new circumstances is an important step in coping with change.
- *Interest*—a shift to concentrating on the potential benefits of change and not just on the potential problems involved.
- *Mental tryout*—this means imagining the new situation or process in some detail, including all the ways in which it will affect you and your life. There is a lot to be said for trying things out in your mind before doing it in real life.

- *Real life practice*—trying it out, perhaps in just a small way. Could you do just a little of whatever change is necessary, without committing yourself to the whole thing, and see how that turns out?

- *Implementation*—actually making the bigger changes and seeing how they work. This is an experimental stage. It does not yet require a commitment to keeping the change. It also allows actual changes you make to be chosen or adapted in the light of their successes or of negative effects.

- *Commitment*—if the change has resulted in an improvement in your quality of life, then you could decide to keep going with it. You will need to continue with it if it is to make a real difference.

- *Integration*—finally, you could make the change an integral part of your normal life. The good news is that if you have successfully got to this stage, you have learned the skills of making change. This will then help you make further changes.

In order to gain the courage to make changes, it can be helpful to think back to changes that you have already made, whether you did this when you were in good health or when you were ill. Can you identify the stages you went through then, and see how this might match up with your present experience? Can you identify the stage you are at now? Understanding the way in which you made a successful change in the past could help you make changes now.

To cope effectively with change, we all need the right mixture of information and resources. All that we have said earlier and will say later about gathering information applies here. What help do you think you need at this moment? Could you get some of it? What could you do to get more of it? What helped you make the previous change? Looking back, what would have made that change easier? How could you get at least some of the help you require? Maybe just talking to someone sympathetic and informed would be useful.

Management of your general health

It can be very easy to be so caught up in your illness that you forget about looking after your general health. All the sensible things that a healthy person would do to look after themselves are still important. Maybe they are even more important now, as you do not want to burden a body already coping with illness with other problems. There is a section later in the book on the 'sensible' things that you should keep on doing.

Changes that just happen with the passage of time are often ignored. Life and illnesses can alter in subtle ways. We all get older, and new problems can crop up just because of ageing. It is important to keep this in mind, and not think that any new problem can automatically be blamed on your illness.

Discipline

Self-management of your illness can be rewarding, but successful self-management also requires a measure of self-discipline. There are bound to be times that you simply get tired of being disciplined. That is, of course, just being human. So if you feel like that, have a little break, but then come back to the things that you know you should do to help yourself. Do not blame yourself too much if you have times like these, and do not panic and conclude that you cannot make the change. Probably the only person who expects you to be perfect is you!

Developing your own self-management plan

With any illness, there are ways in which you can make things better, just as there are things which can make you feel worse. Some of the ways in which you choose to live your life may reduce your symptoms; some may increase them. It is important to get all the information you can about what is likely to help. You may be given very good advice by your family doctor, by a clinic nurse or by your specialist, but that advice will not necessarily address the whole picture of your illness. Sometimes you are left to get on with it by yourself, which may leave you feeling rather isolated and abandoned. It is then even more important to find out for yourself what would be helpful.

In Chapter 3, we suggested sources of information to help you become an 'expert patient'. Some of these will give you more details about the medical aspects of your illness, but most of them could also help you with self-management. We do urge you always to exercise a healthy degree of scepticism. Not all the things that you read or hear will be sound. See if you can check any information you feel a bit dubious about against another, reliable source.

Support groups

You can often get useful information from people experiencing the same illness as you. If there is a national support organization for your particular illness, it may have a lot of useful advice on self-management. It may also be able to give you the contact details for a support group in your area. Such groups vary a lot. Some are very practical and supply information and advice; some may turn out to be more concerned with discussing symptoms. You would have to attend at least one meeting to decide if that group suits you. It can be very inspiring to be able to talk with people suffering in the same way you are and to hear how they cope. At least with such a group you do not need to explain what you have. However, if you have not been ill for very long, you may find it dispiriting or even frightening to meet people who have been ill for much longer or whose symptoms are worse than yours. If you decide that a local group is not for you, that is fine. You do not *have* to be part of such a group.

Do remember that each individual experiences an illness in a slightly different way and may choose to deal with it in a different way. We suggest that you talk with fellow sufferers and with appropriate support groups and then make up your own mind as to what seems to suit you. Just because someone says that they find such-and-such helpful does not mean that it would help you or that you have to try it. For instance, some people go down the route of trying a lot of alternative therapies, some of which they may find helpful. That might be fine for them, but it may not be the best way for you. You have the choice about this.

Expertise from other illnesses

A central theme of this book is that similar problems occur in most long-term illnesses. You may therefore be able to learn things from people with diagnoses quite different from yours. Reading about how other sufferers cope can often be quite informative.

This book

In later sections, we offer suggestions of different ways in which you could help yourself. These sections are organized to cover physical (biological) factors, emotional (psychological) factors and social or interpersonal factors, though the boundaries between these three groups may sometimes be a bit blurred. You may decide to incorporate some of our ideas into your self-management plan.

Self-help books

Books about your own illness or books about long-term illness in gene~ can often be helpful, as long as you are aware that many of them~ written by people describing how they themselves coped, as if th~

the only way. In Appendix 2, we list some books that we think are particularly good.

The Internet

There may well be useful sites and discussion groups for people with your illness. You may already have accessed some of them to find out more about your illness. Many of these also exchange ideas about self-management. Do, however, try to be discerning about any such information. It is not all helpful. You will probably read about a wide range of experiences, but you do need to remember that different people and nationalities experience things differently.

A written plan

Once you have accessed information, you can start to work out your own self-management plan, keeping it flexible enough to cope with such things as flare-ups in your condition. You may find it helpful to write down your plan. As an example:

Frankie's self-management programme for chronic fatigue syndrome

I found it helpful to look at this under the three headings of biological, psychological and social.

Biological

The two symptoms that cause me most difficulty are fatigue and pain. I manage fatigue partly by pacing—stopping any activity *before* I become too tired—and partly by structuring my life so that I use my energy most efficiently. I try to allow for unexpected demands on me. I use relaxation to give me the best quality rest between 'bites' of activity. I do my best to manage my pain using all the things that help a little, rather than relying totally on painkillers, though I do use just enough of them to keep my pain down to a manageable level. I exercise regularly. I have a 10 minute non-aerobic exercise routine worked out for me by a physiotherapist, which I do most mornings. I use the local learner swimming pool two mornings a week, alternating bending and stretching exercises with very gentle swimming. I walk short distances regularly. I stick to a healthy diet and am careful not to put on weight.

Psychological

I recognize that getting exhausted leads to low spirits, which is another reason for pacing myself carefully. I have given myself a 'worry time' during the afternoon, so that if I have problems I do not ruminate about them at other times. Writing is important to me, both as an interesting occupation but also because getting something published is very good for my self-esteem. I still do a small amount of telephone counselling, which I enjoy and which makes me feel needed. If I feel low about some aspect of my life or illness, I write it down, which helps me understand exactly what the problem is. I then often discuss it with my sister.

Social and interpersonal
I find face-to-face social contact for more than a short time can be very tiring, so most of my contacts are on the phone or by e-mail, which is much less tiring. I cherish the friends who understand my situation and who do not ask too much of me. I have built up a list of contacts, whether friends and relations or people that I pay, who can help me with the things I am now unable to do for myself. I am getting older, so I need to plan for the future when I will be able to do less for myself. I want to stay as independent as I can for as long as I can, and not be a burden for my children.

Self-management courses

You may find that there are group courses in self-management that you could join. If you attend a clinic for your particular condition, that clinic may offer such courses. In the UK, there are also courses offered under the Expert Patient Initiative. Some of these are for one specific illness or disease; others cater for people with somewhat similar conditions. There are many similar courses in other countries. (Using the search engine Google, we found pages of suggestions on the Internet.)

Being part of a group working on the same problems you experience can be empowering and very helpful, but some of the courses tackle problems in ways that may not suit you. Use your own judgement about this. Do not despair if there is nothing suitable in your area. It really is possible to do it on your own (with, perhaps, a bit of help from a book like this).

Be prepared to go on learning

You may find that working out what is the best self-management plan for you has to be a matter of trial and error. Be prepared to test things out. Very few people get things absolutely right first time, so be tolerant of yourself if something that you have tried does not seem to be helping. You may find that one of your symptoms is more troublesome than another, so it may help to concentrate on what seems to reduce that, even if only a little. Be prepared to keep on learning.

Your circumstances may change. You could find that one symptom becomes more troublesome or you may develop some other problems. Your management plan may need to be adapted to cope with this. Be prepared to be flexible.

Some examples

You might find it helpful to read about how different people with different illnesses found advice on self-management:

- Katerina is a 50-year-old woman with fairly bad asthma. When she moved house and changed to a new doctor she was told that there was an asthma nurse attached to the practice. This nurse checked that she was using her inhalers correctly, and together they worked out a written plan for controlling her asthma.

- James was 50 years old when his doctor diagnosed him as having type 2 (non-insulin-dependent) diabetes, which could be controlled by the right diet. The doctor gave him advice about such a diet. James also sent off for literature from the British Diabetes Association.

- Beth is an American woman with CFS/ME (CFIDS). She has joined a local self-help group, but she has also taken part in an online self-management course.

- Tom had a heart attack. Though he is now fairly well, he is suffering from depression. He has taken part in a rehabilitation course run by his hospital clinic. He is also getting treatment from a cognitive behavioural therapist, who has helped him identify the negative beliefs and thoughts about having had a heart attack, which are fuelling his depression.

- Melita has psoriasis. She attends a hospital clinic, which has helped her with drugs and advice. She has also searched the web for information, but is discriminating about what advice she follows.

- Ken is HIV positive. He gets advice from his hospital clinic, but he uses his local support group and the Internet to find out about developments in treatment.

Sharing your management plan with those around you

It will make it much easier for you to stick to your management plan if those around you—a partner, family, significant friends—understand what it is and why it is important. To give just one example from the selection above, James needed to involve his wife in his necessary dietary changes as she was the one who cooked for him. She was keen to do what she could to help, but needed information to do so.

6 Keeping going with a self-management programme

Even if you have a self-management programme that you know is really helpful, keeping going with it can be surprisingly difficult, particularly when the first enthusiasm has died away. If you have been getting on-going medical support and that support comes to and end, it can be even more difficult to keep going. This is a common problem.

I find it hard to keep going with some elements of my own self-help programme. Doing an exercise routine every morning can become tedious; getting up on a cold morning to go to the swimming pool can seem very unattractive. It does seem to help that I see my doctor every three months when she asks about how I am managing myself. Keeping reminding myself of the benefits of the programme is also a help. I know that if I stop doing my exercises for more than a few days I get much stiffer and hurt more, as well as beginning to feel unattractively flabby. Another thing that helps is to allow myself a 'holiday' from coping occasionally. For instance, I sometimes give myself a day during which I take more painkillers than usual and don't bother with all the other pain management techniques. Frankie

So what are the things that you might find could help? Here are some suggestions:

- Do not make your programme too rigid. Five or six days a week is probably enough, except for those things that are really medically vital such as sticking to managing diabetes well.
- Give yourself an occasional 'holiday' from coping. You may well find that you come back to the programme the next day feeling refreshed and ready to start again.
- Try to find someone to whom you can report your progress. The idea of a 'buddy' (perhaps someone with the same condition as yourself) you talk to once a week, even if only briefly, can be very helpful in keeping you on track.

- Some kind of medical supervision, even if infrequent, can be useful. You might perhaps be able to negotiate with your doctor for a meeting every 6 months or so, during which you discuss your self-help programme.

- Be very clear in your mind about what are the benefits of sticking to your programme, perhaps less malaise, less pain or fatigue, moving more easily—whatever applies to your particular case. Reminding yourself about what you gain from your programme can help you keep your motivation going.

- Give yourself rewards for sticking to your programme.

- Find ways of making what you need to do less boring. For instance, would you find exercise more fun if you did it in a class, so that you could add in the benefits of social contact?

Finally, do involve anyone you live with in what you are doing. Make certain that they understand what it is and why it is important for you to continue with it.

What gets in the way of being 'sensible'?

Sticking to a management programme in a consistent way is not easy. You may well find that there are a lot of things, some coming from your own thoughts and beliefs and some from external pressures, that get in the way of you managing yourself in the best way—'what gets in the way of being sensible'. This is a very common problem.

There are three main areas in which people slip away from a good management programme—doing too much, doing too little and failing to stick to the medical advice they have been given on such things as medication, diet and exercise. Often these lapses only happen some of the time—for much of the time you can stick to most of your management programme—but it can be helpful for you to notice the circumstances around a lapse. If you understand what things are likely to push you off course, then you will have a very much better chance of being able to do something about it. It often helps if you can catch the fleeting thought just before you do something that is not 'sensible'.

Your beliefs and thoughts

Most people are, to some degree, driven by what are called 'imperatives'; these are thoughts and attitudes that include words such as 'ought', 'must' and 'should'. They commonly reflect beliefs acquired during childhood.

If you think about yourself, you might be able to recognize some 'imperatives' of your own. Typical ones can be:

- If you have started something, you really *ought* to finish it
- You *must* try to do better than that
- You *should* be getting on with things instead of just sitting around doing nothing
- You *ought* not to complain
- You *should* always put other people's needs above your own.

You might even be able to hear the adult voice who said that to the child you used to be and challenge it now. You do need to think about whether certain beliefs are appropriate to the person you are today. They can certainly get in the way of good self-management.

Typical thoughts you can begin to recognize as pointers to 'imperatives' might include:

- I'll just finish the job and then I'll rest
- I know I'm tired, but I do want to get this finished
- People will think I'm being selfish if I don't join in with their plans
- I'm tired of being sensible
- I must look after my family in the way I used to
- It won't matter if I do (or don't do) such-and-such just this once
- Doing such-and such is likely to make me worse
- I'm too ill to do anything
- Maybe I'll harm myself if I do such-and-such.

When and why is self-management difficult?

You will have your own obstacles to effective self-management. In order to give you some ideas though, here are some common ones that people have told us about.

Pressures of just surviving

For a lot of people with a long-term illness—those living on their own, mothers with young children, people with unsupportive families, those struggling to keep on with a job—just doing the minimum to keep going can make over-activity almost unavoidable. It can help if you can stand back and look at all that you believe needs doing and consider whether *some* of it might not be absolutely essential. It might be possible to restructure th▸

way in which the essential is done, breaking tasks down into smaller bites, and stopping for a rest between each one.

Lack of clear management advice

It certainly is a help if you have been given clear medical advice on the best way to manage your particular illness. If a doctor you trust has told you what to do or not do, you will find it much easier to stick to self-management and to explain it to people around you. Unless you have been told that it is safe to stretch yourself a little more, you may play safe and do rather less. If you have not been told to look after yourself, you may do more than is good for you.

Often people get only vague advice, without much information about why a particular behaviour is important. This can make it more difficult to stick to it or explain it to those around you. For instance, sticking to the right diet, especially when you are with other people, is easier if you can say that that is what your doctor has told you to do, and why it matters.

Other people's expectations

It is only too easy to get sucked into doing too much, or behaving in ways that do not suit your illness, by what you believe other people are expecting from you. It is worth considering three things:

1. Are your ideas about their expectations accurate? Could you check up on what they really do want?

2. Are their ideas unreasonable or inaccurate? Could you communicate with them better, so that their ideas are more realistic?

3. How important is it to you to fulfil their expectations? Do you really need to please them if they are being unrealistic?

Your own idea of what makes a 'good person'

We all have a model of a 'good person', which will have been formed over the years, probably starting in childhood. Trying to match up your lifestyle with this model when you are unwell is more than likely to lead you into doing too much or behaving in ways that are not helpful to your condition. It is worth giving some time to thinking about this. Your model may have suited you before you became ill, but does it fit in with the way you are today? Could you work out something more realistic and appropriate? Clinging on to an outdated model could add to your frustration and distress if you cannot match up to it today. The person you are, your 'being', is more important than what you do.

Being a perfectionist

This can be one of the things that really does get in the way of being sensible. If you still believe that everything you do has to be done to a very high standard, you are likely to push yourself far harder than is appropriate for the way you are today, as well as distressing yourself each time you cannot achieve perfection. You may even avoid doing certain things because you know you cannot now do them as well as you used to. Ask yourself:

- Why do I think that I have to be perfect?
- Would I impose such standards on someone else in my circumstances?
- What am I trying to prove and who am I trying to prove it to? This could be stuff from your childhood, which you might be able to set aside today. Perhaps you could try to adopt the motto 'good enough is good enough'.

If you find it hard to shift from being a perfectionist, you might try telling yourself that your self-management programme takes priority and concentrate on doing that in the best way possible.

Not wanting to seem different from the people around you

Particularly in a social situation, it is very understandable that you do not want to behave differently from your friends. You would prefer to join in suggested activities. It can be very hard to say no. For instance, you may find it hard to stick to a recommended diet if it means that you cannot eat the same things as your friends. If you can give a calm and simple explanation of why you need to do, or not do, certain things, it usually gets easier. You do need to watch out for ignorant people who say things like 'It won't do you any harm just this once'.

Pride

Many people find that pride gets in the way of good management. They resent asking for help or feel that they would be less of a person if they dropped their standards. Asking for help does not make you less of a person; high standards probably do not matter quite as much as you think they do. Consider the difference between pride and self-respect. Self-respect is important; pride is not.

Fear

Fear can get in the way of good self-management. It is often so hard to be certain about what could help and what could harm, particularly if you have one of the illnesses with no medically explained cause and if you have not been given authoritative advice. It can be difficult to be certain how much you could safely do. It can be tempting to avoid activity for fear of making yourself worse. We hope that this book will help you understand more about what is possible and safe.

If you did something and felt very unwell afterwards, you can quite justifiably feel nervous about trying it again. However, it could be that you did too much of it or you did it at a time when you were already tired from doing something else. That activity might be within your capacity now if you timed it better or did it for a shorter time.

Even if you have an illness with a clear diagnosis, such as arthritis or heart disease, you may still be fearful of some activities, thinking that they may cause more pain or might damage you in some way. Do discuss this with your doctor or specialist, and get reassurance that it is safe to push yourself a little more, and that the recommended activity, far from being harmful, would actually be helpful.

It is not only the sufferer who can be fearful. Partners and carers can sometimes hold a person back. If you are asked questions such as 'Should you be doing such-and-such? Are you sure that it's safe?' it might be a sign that they care, but it might also show that they are being rather too controlling. You may need to get your doctor to talk with them and explain that such activities are safe and beneficial.

The 'sick person' role

Inactivity can be as bad for you as over-activity. Keeping yourself as active as possible under the circumstances is often not easy, but it can be very important both for your body and for your quality of life. There may well be times when you have to resist pressure from those around you to do less. Family and friends may feel that they should express how much they care by doing as much as they can for you. 'Poor darling, let me do that for you'. If you are in that position, try to find ways of explaining to them that doing things for yourself is important to you. You are not rejecting them if you reject some of their help.

You are more than just your illness. Behaving most of the time as if your illness has to shape your entire life will diminish you and will certainly reduce the amount of pleasure you can experience.

Being ill can be depressing and depression can sap your motivation, so that it seems hardly worth the bother of doing things. If you recognize that this is a problem for you, then see if you can get help. Setting yourself small targets, and getting satisfaction from achieving them, will be a boost to your morale.

Not acknowledging the limitations of your illness—rejecting the 'sick person' role—can lead you astray too. You may use your body in ways that do it no good at all.

Acceptance and denial

Following up from the last point, one of the things that can make sensible self-management more difficult can be not accepting the realities that your condition imposes—being in denial. People tend to talk as if acceptance was a one-off, finite, 'boom, boom, I've got there' kind of thing. It is not. It has to be a constant process of adjustment. Probably nobody accepts all their limitations all of the time.

Accepting the realities of your illness does not mean that you have given in to it or given up, rather the reverse. Being realistic gives you a better chance of managing your condition and getting the best quality of life in the circumstances. It certainly does not mean that you have to like what you are going through.

Acceptance has to be a dynamic, not a static process. Each day is likely to bring new challenges, emotional and physical, to which you need to adapt. The tension between acceptance and denial is always there. You may have to accept three different possibilities—you could improve, you could stay much the same or you could deteriorate—and keep an open mind about all three, while dealing the best you can with what is happening today.

If your condition is deteriorating, then each downward slide can bring new restrictions that could be accepted or denied. If tomorrow may bring extra difficulties and burdens, then it can be quite allowable to give yourself short periods of respite during which you assume/pretend that tomorrow will be OK or at least not worse. This is not the same as denial, more like a therapeutic break. If this is something you recognize in yourself, do your best not to get stuck in the mode of not thinking about the future at all. Sensible planning, so that you have an idea about how you could cope with a less that favourable tomorrow, can be very helpful.

Doctors and family may suggest that you should 'come to terms' with your illness, as if it was a one-off thing. You know better. Just keep working on accepting at least some of what is happening today.

Looking at what you are getting right

So far, we have looked at some of the things that may get in the way of you managing yourself in the best way, and suggested that you identify the factors particular to your own situation. Another approach to good management is to identify the times and the circumstances in which you do stick to your management programme. What is the difference? Thinking about this may help you modify your thinking or your behaviour in ways that would help you to be more consistent. In any case, giving yourself credit for your successes would be good for your self-esteem.

7 Using complementary/ alternative medicine (CAM)

One way of managing a long-term illness that you may consider is to use complementary or alternative therapies. These are treatments that lie outside conventional medicine. The distinction between complementary and alternative can be somewhat blurred. Complementary therapies tend to be those that it is suggested are used alongside conventional medicine. Indeed, some doctors have trained in some of these treatments such as homeopathy and acupuncture. Alternative therapies (as the name suggests), on the other hand, are more likely to be suggested as an alternative to conventional treatment. These therapies can range from things that your doctor might be happy to recommend to some that are frankly bizarre and possibly dangerous.

Such therapies are being used by more and more of us. It is not surprising that many people with a long-term illness make use of such therapies alongside their normal medical treatment. Some therapies are well established and can be very helpful; others can be less so. Though there is now some research being carried out into some therapies, benefits are often uncertain. However, the fact that so many people continue to use both complementary and alternative therapies, even though they may not lead to any reduction in symptoms, suggests that they are getting *something* from them. There may be benefits that are less easy to quantify such as a feeling of being cared for.

It is sometimes suggested that any benefits from a complementary/ alternative therapy are due more to the therapeutic effect of the patient– therapist relationship rather than to any specific treatment. This could be possible. Any patient can tell you that having a good relationship with a doctor or a therapist is potentially powerful. Some sceptics may say 'It's *only* a placebo'. Why *only* a placebo? Look back at what we said about the placebo effect in Chapter 3. Though doctors may not understand the mechanism, it is a real effect.

Potential benefits of trying any treatment

- CAM may appeal to you as being more 'natural' than mainstream medicine.

- A CAM therapist may give you more time than a busy doctor is able to offer. Just having someone listening to your problems in a sympathetic way and taking an interest in you as a person (not just as a case) can be helpful. On-going support can make managing any illness much easier.

- You may prefer to be able to choose a treatment for yourself rather than having it decided for you by a doctor.

- You may find it helpful.

- The idea that you are doing something to help yourself may give you a sense of control over your illness.

- Any reduction in symptoms, even if limited or temporary, is to be welcomed.

Potential disadvantages of trying any treatment

- In general, complementary/alternative therapists are subject to less regulation than doctors. There is, therefore, more opportunity for dubious treatment and unethical practice.

- If you do improve, you may mistakenly give the credit to the therapy or therapist rather than to what you are doing to help yourself or to the natural progress of the condition. This may reduce your feeling of being able to manage your illness yourself. You may also feel that continued improvement depends on continuing with the treatment.

- If the therapy does not do you any good, having your expectations of improvement disappointed may add to your feelings of frustration and hopelessness.

- It may cost you a lot of money (which might be better spent on other things).

- If there is no improvement, some therapists may blame the patient— saying that they have not tried hard enough or persisted long enough. While this may sometimes be true, life with a long-term illness can be tough enough without being blamed in this way.

- You may find that your doctor is very dismissive of your use of such therapies, and your pursuit of them may affect the relationship between the two of you.

Why do you want a treatment?

This may seem like a silly question to ask, but people do have very different reasons for seeking treatment. If you are clear in your mind about what you want from the treatment, it will help you choose.

- Are you looking for a 'cure'? Do you believe that if you go on looking long enough you will find one? The plain truth is that this is very unlikely. If this is your hope, then you are probably heading for disappointment.
- Are you looking for something that will make you feel better generally, such as a reduction in symptoms? Would you like something that is helpful or pleasurable, even in the short term?
- Are you looking for help with one or more specific symptoms?
- Are you looking for an increase in energy and an improvement in what you are able to do?
- Are you looking for support and encouragement?
- Are you unhappy that you are not being offered any treatment for your condition?

Sensible precautions

If you do decide to try a complementary/alternative therapy, there are some questions you should ask the therapist. You have a right to question anyone offering treatment before you agree to it. You do not need to be hesitant or embarrassed about this.

- What does the treatment offer? Does it match what you want from it? What evidence is there that this treatment has a good chance of doing this? Has there been any good-quality research on the treatment?
- Has the therapist got experience of using this treatment in patients with your particular illness? If so, how many? What results has he or she had with them? Does he or she understand the problems you have?
- What are the risks of side effects or even of being made worse with this treatment?
- What training and qualifications does the therapist have? (It is not always easy to judge how worthwhile these are for some CAM therapists.) What does the training involve? How long does it take?
- Does the therapist belong to a professional organization that monitors training and standards of treatment? (Again this is not always easy to

judge.) Can that organization enforce standards? Is there a complaints procedure?

- How long is the treatment likely to last? Does the therapist insist on a minimum number of treatments and, if so, why? (Be cautious about this one.)
- If you are paying for the treatment, how much is it going to cost in total (including tests, drugs, etc.)? Think about what you might have to give up in order to afford it. Would you do better spending that money on something that makes your life easier or gives you pleasure?
- What would the cost be in terms of your energy? Would you have to travel to have the treatment? Would the fatigue of getting there and back as well as having the treatment outweigh any benefits?
- Does the therapist carry proper professional insurance?
- Will the therapist keep in touch with your usual doctor?

Monitoring results

If you do decide to try a therapy, you need to monitor if it is helping and how much in order to decide whether to continue. This is why we suggest that you are clear about what you want from it. You may need to try more than just one treatment or continue with a herbal remedy or supplement for a while before you can judge its effectiveness. The therapist should be able to advise you how long it will be before you could expect to see a result. If, after taking this into account, you feel worse or it does not seem to be helping, then you have a right to stop. As a rough guide, if you cannot see any significant benefit after 6 weeks, it would probably be better to stop. Do not let yourself be bullied into continuing if you do not want to. Give yourself a pause. You can then decide whether to continue or to try something else. If you are paying for the treatment, you may decide to use the money in a different way.

We are certainly not in a position to recommend any particular therapies. This is something you have to decide for yourself, but you might well find that the right therapy for you does offer some benefits. Talking with other people who suffer from the same illness as you do could be useful in deciding whether to try something. A personal recommendation can be helpful, as long as you remember that no one experiences an illness in exactly the same way, and no one responds to medication and/or therapy in exactly the same way.

Further information

The Which? Guide to Complementary Medicine.

section 2
Managing physical/biological problems

8 Managing fatigue

Fatigue is one of the most common symptoms of many long-term illnesses. It can range from just getting tired more easily than normal to a feeling of total exhaustion after not doing much. It can reduce your activities and take the edge off your pleasure in what you do manage. As this is probably one of the three or four symptoms that most reduces quality of life, it seems reasonable to start a discussion of managing specific problems with this one.

Although we cannot suggest a 'magic bullet' of a drug that will eliminate fatigue, we can suggest ways of managing it. If you tire easily and have a very limited amount of energy, then it is very important to manage what energy you do have in the best way so that you are able to do more without becoming exhausted. There are various techniques that really do help.

Discuss this problem with your doctor

It is always worth mentioning this problem to your doctor. He or she can check for other things apart from your illness that might be factors. For instance, you might be anaemic (a well known cause of fatigue) or the drugs you are taking might cause fatigue as a side effect. Pain and/or sleep problems may be adding to your difficulties. Your diet may be poor, which can add to fatigue. There may be things your doctor can suggest that would help.

Pacing

You may find this helpful. Pacing means balancing time-limited periods of activity, both physical and mental, with periods of good quality rest. It involves stopping when you are only a little tired, rather than going on until you are exhausted. If you break your activities into short 'bites', and rest between bites, you are likely to find that you do not get nearly so tired and that you achieve rather more. Most people who suffer fatigue find that mental activity can be as tiring as physical, so something like sitting down to watch television may not be particularly restful.

It is easy enough to say 'do things in small bites' but that does involve a good deal of discipline and may mean changing the way you used to do things, which can be very hard at first. You may take some time to get into the swing of it. At first, you may well find it frustrating to not be able to finish off a task in one go; leaving something half done and coming back to it later may seem very unnatural to you. It can be very tempting to just keep going until some job is complete or to get carried away and not notice until too late just how tired you have got. Some people find it helps to use a kitchen timer for some tasks, set for a period that they know from experience they can manage comfortably. Once you have mastered this technique though, the reduction of symptoms and an increase in what you can achieve in total can be very rewarding.

You may feel that only being able to do one particular thing for a short time means that you cannot achieve anything major. That is not an accurate belief. A lot of 'small bites' can add up to something significant. For instance, much of this book and our previous one were written by Frankie using the computer for only half an hour most days.

The other aspect of pacing is spreading activities evenly though the day and through the week. Doing most things in the morning and then spending the afternoon feeling exhausted is going to make you feel worse and you will probably achieve less. Scheduling two major events on consecutive days can be a mistake. It is better if you try to give yourself a quiet time before and after a day when you know you will have to do rather more than usual.

Using relaxation

Relaxation, both physical and mental, can be a helpful tool in the management of many aspects of your illness, including fatigue. So what do we mean by relaxation? We do not mean just 'taking it easy', but rather a deliberate letting go of tension in all your muscle groups whilst keeping your mind calm. The most effective rest between periods of activity can come when you are truly relaxed. It can make a difference in the management of pain. It can help you get to sleep, or rest comfortably when you cannot sleep. It is also one of the ways in which you can deal better with stress.

There are many books and tapes available to guide you in the technique. (We suggest some in Appendix 2.) There may be classes available locally, perhaps offered by your hospital clinic. You may already be familiar with the technique, perhaps from studying yoga or from Natural Childbirth classes, though needing to brush up your skills. However you choose to learn, accept that it takes time and practice to be able to do it really well. Do not expect to be perfect right away.

Relaxation is a skill that needs to be practised regularly. Do not think that just mastering the technique is enough. Set aside at least 15 minutes every day for practice. As you get more skilful, you will find that you are able to relax even when you are not lying down. If you are about to do something stressful, such as making a difficult phone call, it helps to give yourself a minute or two during which you drop your shoulders, breathe calmly and relax as much of your body as possible. It is a good idea to check on your state of tension or relaxation regularly during the day.

How to start learning to relax

Choose a time and a place where you will not be disturbed. Make yourself comfortable, whether lying down or sitting in a chair that gives you good support, in a quiet, warm room. Some people find it easier if the room is dark. Loosen your clothing—take off your tie or undo your belt.

It is easy enough to say 'relax your muscles', but it can be quite hard to achieve if you have not learned and practised the techniques. If this is new to you, one of the best ways to start is to learn to recognize the difference between tense and relaxed. Take a few calm breaths, deliberately tense up just one part of your body, and then let it go. Think of different muscle groups, and see how each one feels when you have let go. It is not necessary to do this every time, or do it for every part of your body at one time, but it can be a help at the beginning.

You could try beginning with one arm. See that it is comfortably supported, clench your fist for a moment, and then let it relax. Think about your hand, wrist and forearm getting warmer and heavier, so that if someone were to lift your arm by your cuff, you would let them do it without trying to help, and when they let go, your arm would flop back. Try it again with the other arm. Having mastered that, focus your attention on other parts of your body, and relax different muscle groups in the same way. Many people are particularly tense in their shoulders and neck, so that is an area to concentrate on. It is very important to keep checking on your face. If you are frowning or clenching your teeth, then the rest of your body is likely to be tense as well. Try to smooth your forehead and keep a calm and peaceful expression. Let your lips and tongue relax. You do not have to let your mouth drop open, but do keep your teeth from touching.

A more sophisticated version of relaxation allows you to keep most of your body relaxed even when one muscle group is being used. You can practise this by deliberately tensing up one arm or one leg while you work at keeping the rest of your body relaxed.

Calm breathing

Calm breathing is an important component of relaxation. Slow breathing that uses your ribs and diaphragm, rather than hurried gasps using just the top of your chest, will help you feel peaceful and be good for your body. Breathing out fully is probably more important than concentrating on breathing in (if you have breathed out fully, breathing in will be automatic). If you find this difficult, you may be able to get help with the problem from a physiotherapist.

Relax your mind

You will get much more benefit from relaxation if you are not fretting or worrying over a problem. Postpone that to another time. The ideal is a calm mind in a calm body. Achieving such a peaceful mental state can often be hard, but it does get easier with practice. Find something calm and pleasant to think about, which can replace the worrying thoughts. Many of the relaxation tapes available have suitable visualizations or gentle music. Some people like to think of a special place, one they know well or one they have imagined, and think about all the details of it. Think of this place as a sanctuary you can visit whenever you choose. If worrying thoughts come into your head, acknowledge them and then move back to thinking about your sanctuary.

Meditation

Many people find benefit from combining relaxation with the techniques of meditation. There are different versions—transcendental meditation, mindfulness meditation and Buddhist meditation to name just three. You may need to experiment to find just what suits you. We give details of some books on the subject in Appendix 2. There may be classes or groups in your area which you could join. It is often helpful to practise in company.

After relaxation

Take time to move slowly out of your state of relaxation. Take a few more calm breaths and then stretch a little. Think about how a cat stretches luxuriously before it gets up. Enjoy the ease of body you have achieved.

Possible problems

Not everyone enjoys practising relaxation. You may find that at first you notice pain or malaise more when you are not being distracted by activity, which can be worrying. Just accept that things are not actually worse—you are just noticing them more. That is one of the reasons why 'busying your mind with quietude' can be so important. You may feel a little guilty that you are not 'doing'. Keep hold of the idea that by relaxing you are doing something very important in managing your illness.

An activity diary

When you start a pacing programme, it can be a great help to keep an activity diary for a *few* weeks in which you record activities, timings, symptoms and emotions. (Try using a notebook with one page for each day, and four columns on each page.) After you have kept a record for a while, you will probably be able to spot patterns, such as the swings between doing too much and too little. The diary will give you insights into the activities that are particularly tiring. (You may find that you are surprised by some of the results.) It can help you plan out a 'programme' of balanced rest and activity. It will also help you judge what is the appropriate 'bite size' for different activities. Another useful piece of information could be the correlation between your state of fatigue and your emotions.

Budgeting your energy

When we talk about energy, we do not mean motivation, the desire to get something done. What we do mean is something more like the scientific definition of energy—'the capacity for, the ability to do work'. Managing a limited amount of energy can be rather like managing a low income. If you have not got much money, you need to think about what you spend your money on, and not fritter any of it away. In the same way, you need to think carefully about what you are doing to make the most of what energy you have got. A structured way to think about it can be under these headings.

What are you doing and *why* are you doing it?

It can be helpful to keep a diary of all your activities for a week or two. Is all you do essential? Does it all have to be done by you? Could you encourage other people in the household to share some of the tasks?

Obviously, some of the things you do are essential, but people often realize that they do other things just because that is what they have always done, or because they are pressured into it by other people.

How are you doing it and *when* are you doing it?

You could try standing back and looking at how you do things. Imagine that you had a time and motion expert watching you. What suggestions would such an expert make? Could you do things in a more efficient, labour-saving way? Could you plan things better to cut out unnecessary movement? For instance, could you rearrange things in the kitchen so that you can reach the things you use most often without having to move far? It is always a good idea to pause for a moment's thought before starting anything. Could you invest in a few pieces of equipment that would make things easier? Even a more efficient can opener might be a help.

It helps if you notice the pattern of when you do things. Could you plan things a little better so that you spread out what you do during the day and during the week?

All this does not just apply to household tasks. The same methods can be used in other aspects of your life. You may still be working, but finding it very tiring. There may be ways in which you could make your work easier. You could perhaps structure short rest periods into your day, even if it is just sitting back, closing your eyes and relaxing for a few minutes. Equally, you could think about structuring your social activities in a rather different way so that you do not get exhausted by them.

Pleasure is a vital part of your 'diet'. It is just as important as good food. It needs to be built into your programme. You do not have to feel guilty about using some of your energy on doing the things that give you pleasure or satisfaction (and you should resist pressure from other people to concentrate only on chores). Pleasure is very good for you.

A gradual increase in your activity

Once you have got into a good pacing routine, it is likely that you could feel able to do a little more, but it is important to make any increases gradually. Being too ambitious could set you back. For instance, if you are at present comfortable with doing one particular thing for 10 minutes, you could try the experiment of increasing it to 11 or 12 minutes. Another way would be to do it for 6 minutes, but then repeat it later in the day. A very small increase may seem to be insignificant but, when repeated, such increases can add up to something very significant. Beware of judging yourself against what you used to be able to do. What you are able to do now is what matters.

With all increases, it is helpful to think about some very definite targets. Instead of thinking something like 'I'd like to be able to walk much further', try replacing that rather vague aim with something much more specific like 'I'd like to be able to walk to the park and back'. Then think about building up to that distance in stages over several weeks. We talk more about this kind of goal setting in Chapter 15.

Choosing your priorities

If what you are able to do is limited by lack of energy or by other symptoms, you are not going to be able to do everything. You have to make choices. Take time to think about all the things that you want to do (or feel you ought to do), and then pick out what is most important to you. There are bound to be things that you would like to do, but which have to be set aside in favour of other things that matter more. For instance, if you are still working, you may need to cut back on your social life a bit.

Be gentle with yourself

This sort of discipline is not easy, particularly at the beginning. You do not have to be perfect at it. We can all make mistakes, and we need to be forgiving of ourselves when we do. Often we can learn a lot from getting things a bit wrong. It can be hard at first, but it does get easier with practice. Sticking too rigidly to a pacing programme can be demoralizing. Give yourself a holiday from it sometimes, as long as it is not too often and not for too long.

Think about what you find most tiring

Start to notice which things tire you more than others. They will not necessarily be physical activities. (There may also be things that cause you more pain—see Chapter 9.) Many people find that mental activities or stressful situations can be even more exhausting. Could you get help with specific tasks or find a way to make them easier? Stress is such an important topic that we talk about it more in Chapter 21.

Asking for help

This can often be difficult. If you were a self-sufficient person before you became ill, then having to delegate tasks to others may seem very unnatural. We have found that many people find it very difficult to ask for help. We talk more about this in Chapter 24. It is worth thinking about how you could overcome your reluctance.

Managing mental fatigue

Mental activity can often be as tiring as physical activity—sometimes even more so. If you know that you tire easily, you may have to make choices about the proportion of your time that you spend on each of them.

You may need to think about just how much you value your mental activity as opposed to your physical activity. If the way you use your brain is important to you, then you may need to 'ration' how much you do physically so that you can enjoy more of mental activities.

You may find that, when you are tired, you have more difficulty concentrating or find it hard to remember some things. Try not to let this worry you—it is very unlikely to be the onset of dementia! Once you have rested, you will find that your mental abilities return.

There is a lot that you can do to help yourself, both in propping up a poor memory and in doing small things to maintain cognitive function:

- Cut down on what you absolutely have to remember.
- Use lists. Write things down. It can be helpful to use a notebook or something like a Filofax or an electronic equivalent, so that you know where you have made the note—you can waste a lot of time and effort trying to remember on which scrap of paper you wrote the information.
- Try to build up routines to help you remember things—such as always putting the car keys in the same place immediately after you come into the house.
- Give yourself a few moments before you do something to get it clear in your head.
- Take time to consider what gives you the greatest difficulty and then think about practical ways to make things easier.

With something that really does need to be remembered, you can experiment with different ways of learning it. Writing it down, saying it out loud, using word association, and so on can all make something easier to capture.

If you have difficulty concentrating, try doing the things that require concentration in much smaller 'bites'. Just do part of a task, have a rest, and then come back to it later. Cut out distractions such as noise or conversation. Choose a time of day when concentration seems a little easier to do the demanding tasks. One of the tasks that people can find the most difficult and stressful is filling in official forms. Allow yourself to tackle them slowly, perhaps doing just one page or one section a day. Forcing yourself to go on until the job is finished may be very tiring and will probably mean that you do it much less efficiently. A warning note—putting off the difficult task will often mean that you face a deadline and then need to do it in a hurry. Try to start in good time.

Keeping in practice with mental activities

It is well worth keeping in regular practice with mental activities you find difficult. If you give up bothering with something because it is difficult, it is likely to get worse because you are out of practice. To a degree, it is a case of 'use it or lose it'. Your brain needs exercise just as your body does. Quite simple things can help a lot. To give just one example, if you have difficulty in finding the right word (which is something we often hear about), doing just a little of a very simple crossword can be a good therapy.

9 Managing pain

Living with pain can be especially hard. Pain may be a constant background to your life, or it may be intermittent, perhaps made worse by activity. It can be a very lonely experience too; pain is not visible to other people, who can probably never understand just what it is like for you. Pain can be very tiring in itself, as well as interfering with your sleep. It can get in the way of things you want to do. We do not believe that 'what can't be cured must be endured'. We do believe that it can be managed. Anything that you can do to manage your pain—to reduce it or to lessen its impact—will be a help to your body and to your mind. There really are things that you can do that will help.

Some pain has a clear cause that can be diagnosed by your doctor, and for which there may be treatments that can help to some degree. However, a surprising number of people suffer pain with no clear disease cause. This does not mean that there is no physical cause, or that the pain is not real, but that it is just not something that doctors can identify by the tests they have available. This can be very hard for the person suffering such pain, who can be left with no label for their suffering and no treatment. Some people may even suggest that the pain is 'psychological', which may be seen as implying that it is imagined or even your own fault, a particularly upsetting accusation.

Some such sufferers embark on a long, and usually fruitless, quest for someone, somewhere, who will be able to provide the elusive disease diagnosis and a curative treatment. In fact, pain often continues long after the original injury has gone. This is because of changes in the brain and spinal cord, which continue to register pain.

It can be very hard to give up the hope of finding a definite disease cause for your pain and a cure for it, and instead to settle down to looking at what you could do yourself to manage it. Perhaps the answer for you is to work at pain management, while being aware of the possibility that a new piece of evidence might emerge that could suggest a diagnosis and maybe a treatment.

What you can do to help yourself

Though there is a definite place for the use of drugs to ease pain, most people who suffer long-term pain find that there are also other things that help. You are probably using some of these strategies already, but it is always a good idea to extend your range. We can offer you a variety of suggestions for managing your own pain but, as with so much of what we recommend, you will have to experiment to find what works for you. We realize that, if we are talking about long-term illness in general, that covers a very wide range of different kinds and degrees of pain. What works for one person and one condition will not necessarily work for another person or condition. Some of the things that you try may not help much, but, after all, any reduction of pain is to be welcomed. Several little changes can together make a big difference.

Taking control of your life by using self-management of the pain will make you feel more in control and less helpless. You do not need to choose between drugs or self-management; you could use both.

Do not assume that all your pain is due to the disease you have

Be prepared to consider that there may be other causes for *some* of your pain. Discuss this with your family doctor or your specialist. Make sure that other conditions that could cause pain have been considered and treated. For example:

- Chronic pain can lead to depression, and depression can worsen pain. Treating the depression can reduce the pain.
- A sedentary life can cause back and joint pain, which might be relieved by appropriate exercise.
- Drug withdrawal can cause headaches.
- Onset of degenerative arthritis can cause pain.

Being sensible about looking at additional causes for your pain can be helpful; continually searching for a main cause is not.

Long-term illness involves the passage of time. The ageing process continues for all of us. Things change and new problems may crop up. You will need to allow for this and consider adapting your self-management programme.

Relaxation and meditation

Pain can cause muscle tension and also be made worse by it. For instance, some headaches are the result of tension in the neck and shoulders. Try the effect of relaxing in response to pain, rather than tightening up against it. You may well find that deep relaxation, especially in the muscle groups around the site of the pain, will ease things considerably. This is particularly true of abdominal pain. Regular, daily practice will make it easier to move into a relaxed mode when you need it. Calm, slow breathing will also help. The effects may be short term, but moments of respite are to be welcomed.

A lot of people find that meditation combined with relaxation can help. There is research evidence that the techniques of mindfulness meditation can help pain sufferers. If you have a calm mind in a calm body, it can be easier to cope with pain.

Distraction

Pain always feels more severe when we are focusing our attention on it. Focusing attention is like shining a searchlight on the sensation. The more we concentrate on it, the worse it may seem. Distraction (concentrating on something else other than your pain, taking your mind off it) can reduce your awareness of your pain, even if you can only keep it up for a few minutes at a time. Again, any moments of respite are to be welcomed.

Once you have got yourself relaxed, try moving on to focusing your awareness on something else. You will need to experiment to find out what works best for you. It could be music, a talking book, an interesting programme on the radio or television, or a pleasant conversation with a friend or relative. It could be concentrating on something that really interests you. You could try thinking of something pleasant and relaxing, such as remembering a place you enjoyed, and concentrating on all the details of sight, sound and smell associated with that place. Sometimes concentrating on a bit of your body that is *not* hurting, even if it is just your little finger, will help. If you use this technique regularly, you may well be able to extend the periods during which you do not notice the pain so much.

Pacing

For many people, going on too long with one particular activity increases pain. We discussed pacing in Chapter 8 as a help in managing fatigue, but this concept can also be applied to pain management. One of the techniques used in specialized Pain Management Clinics is to time just how long a patient can do one particular activity before pain increases. The patient is then taught to continue the activity for only 80% of that time. It can be very helpful if you can work this out for all the things you do and learn to stop before you reach the point of increased pain. For instance, if you have found that you can do such-and-such for 10 minutes before you start to hurt more, you could make a point of stopping after only 8 minutes, then having a rest or changing to a different activity.

Exercise

Exercise can have an important place in the self-management of pain. *Some* of your pain could be a consequence of lack of activity in illness or poor posture. This is likely to be an added factor if you lead a very sedentary life or spend a lot of time in bed. Muscles that are not used much get weaker; joints get stiff like rusty hinges. When they are used they hurt. You could try a minimal exercise routine to stretch and strengthen your muscles and to keep your joints mobile (as in Chapter 10). Good posture may help to prevent some of these problems.

Depending on your particular disease, it may well be helpful to do specific exercises to strengthen the muscles round a painful joint or to improve the muscle tone in various parts of your body. You may be offered help and advice by your doctor or clinic. You could also try consulting a physiotherapist, a chiropractor, an osteopath or an experienced Pilates or Alexander Technique instructor who could design an exercise routine tailor-made for you. Exercises that strengthen your back will help to avoid future problems.

Getting a little fitter by exercising will probably increase the amount you are able to do and so improve the quality of your life.

Other techniques

It is worth experimenting with all the other things that help just a little, and use them alongside the other management techniques we have discussed. Here are just a few suggestions:

- *Warmth*—do you hurt less if you are warm? Maybe putting a hot-water bottle, or one of the wheat bags that can be heated in a microwave, in the right place would help. An electric blanket in your bed, or an electric pad while you are sitting in a chair, might make a difference. Warm baths do not have to be just for washing—a soak in a bath, or sitting under a hot shower can sometimes ease a sore body and be a pleasantly relaxing experience.

- *Cold*—for some pain, cold is the answer. A gel bag cooled in the refrigerator or a wheat bag cooled in the freezer can help with inflamma-tion, though you should be careful not to use either of them for too long (probably not more than 15 minutes), and never apply them to bare skin—always wrap the bag up.

- *Massage*—the right kind of massage can help some pain. You need to experiment to find what works for you. Sometimes a very light, delicate stroking of the skin above the painful place can be nice and a distraction from the pain. Perhaps you could train a partner or a friend to do massage for you if you cannot afford professional help.

• *Visualization*—you may find that visualization can help. Some people can form a picture of their pain in their minds. If you are one of them, you could experiment with trying to change the picture into something less aggressive (like changing the image of a tiger into one of a gentle kitten). If you think of the pain in a colour, you could try changing that colour to something softer and more friendly. Whatever the picture, try to make it a more positive one.

TENS (transcutaneous electrical nerve stimulation)

TENS machines can be effective for some people, at least for some of their pain, particularly if it is fairly localized. They have the benefit of having no side effects (unlike conventional painkillers). They work by delivering a very small, controlled electrical impulse through electrodes on the skin, which can block the pain message in the nerve. They also stimulate the production of endorphins, the body's own painkillers. They are not cheap. (In the UK they cost £40–£60, but you can get one on approval for 3 weeks, so you could try it out before having to pay for it. With back-up from a doctor or physiotherapist, you may be able to avoid paying VAT.)

Complementary therapies

Some patients report that complementary therapies can sometimes help with some of their pain. For a start, such therapists can usually give more time to a patient than overstretched health professionals. You would also be likely to see the same therapist on repeat visits, which may not be possible with a family doctor or in a hospital clinic. This can be comforting. The evidence from clinical trials for most of these therapies is lacking. Nevertheless, some people report that treatments such as chiropractic, osteopathy, homeopathy, reflexology, acupuncture, shiatsu or aromatherapy have been helpful to them, though others have found that these did not do anything for them. If you can afford such treatment, in terms of both money and energy expenditure, it might be worth experimenting. However, do not allow yourself to feel pressurized by other people into using these therapies, or seduced by the idea that someone else can 'do it all for you'. If you do use such therapies, do not let that stop you going on with self-management techniques. In Chapter 7, we discussed this subject further and offered some suggestions as to what questions to ask of a therapist.

Specialist pain clinics

You may be able to get a referral to a Pain Management Clinic. Such clinics are staffed by professionals who understand pain and the problems pain causes. They look at all the ways in which your pain might be reduced, and offer good advice about what you could do to help yourself. They often practise a holistic approach and can also help with the very strong emotions that long-term pain can evoke.

Managing the emotions that come with pain

The way you think about your pain and your beliefs about it can have an effect on how you cope. Being in pain much of the time can produce very strong emotions such as anger, frustration, resentment, worry, fear and low spirits. All of these can make you focus much more on the pain and reduce your quality of life. Anything that you can do, or can be helped to do, to manage and reduce these emotions will be helpful. We talk more about this in a later section of the book, but here is a brief run through.

Anger

Anger in response to pain is understandable, but it often makes things worse. You may feel angry with your doctors for not being able to cure your pain, or even for not being able to explain why you have it. If your pain began after some trauma, such as a road accident, then you may be angry with the person responsible for the accident. You may simply feel that it is so unfair that you should have to suffer like this—'what did I ever do to deserve this?' People around you who do not seem to understand what you are suffering or be sympathetic can also be the focus of your rage. Frustration at the limitations imposed by pain and resentment at what is happening can add to your anger.

Being stuck in old anger is tiring. It causes tension which can increase pain. It can make it very difficult for the people around you and make it harder for them to help you. You may need expert help with this problem, but just talking about it to someone sympathetic and putting your feelings into words can be a useful start. Writing down your feelings can often help.

Fear and anxiety

Long-term pain is different from short-term pain. Short-term pain mostly has a biological value of warning. Long-term pain is different and does not usually mean that you have anything to fear, as long as you have been checked over by your doctor.

One of the beliefs that many people share is that pain is always a danger signal and so to be feared. This may have been true earlier in your illness or before you became ill, but it is not necessarily so now. Just because doing something causes you pain, does not necessarily mean that that activity is dangerous. Hurt does not always mean harm. You may believe something like 'I mustn't do such-and-such. It hurts, so I must be damaging myself.' This could restrict your life unnecessarily. Take expert advice from your doctor or specialist about what is safe for you to do.

Take a look at what you believe that your pain means. Do you fear that it is a signal that you have some very serious, perhaps even life-threatening, condition? You do not have to be ashamed to admit this—we have heard such fears voiced by very many of the sufferers we have talked to. Discuss it with your doctor and get reassurance.

Inevitably, you may have fears and anxiety about the progression of your illness and the possibility of an increase of pain, which can be hard to deal with. You should not blot out the possibility, but neither should you dwell on it too much. Come back into today, and deal with today. If you are dealing well with today, you are very likely to be able to deal well with tomorrow, no matter what that brings.

Fear is a distressing and demoralizing experience and it is exhausting too. It is bad enough hurting without suffering fear as well, so it is worth looking at the meanings you give to your pain, the labels you put on it, and checking on their accuracy. The more that you can reduce the feelings of fear and resentment of pain, the better it will be for your body and for you. Fear and anger are stressful, and stress can make pain worse, as can tension caused by them. Anything that you can do to reduce these emotions will help.

Low spirits and depression

Being in pain can be a miserable experience, so it is not surprising if you sometimes feel pretty low. Finding ways of having pleasure, in spite of the pain, will help. However, surveys have shown that at least a quarter of people in long-term pain also suffer from true depression. This is something that could and should be treated. Depression can add to your physical pain and make it more difficult for you to manage it. It can certainly reduce your quality of life. There is no reason to be ashamed of it, or to think that it shows lack of moral fibre. Do talk to your doctor and ask for help. In Chapter 22 we talk about the different treatments for depression.

'Painkillers'

Like all medicines, painkillers (analgesic medication) have advantages and disadvantages. You would need to balance the benefits of any pain reduction against side effects. It is worth trying other strategies of managing pain, such as we have outlined earlier, to use alongside such drugs. One fact that needs to be pointed out is that the word 'painkillers' is inaccurate. They very seldom 'kill' pain; they just reduce it.

Depending on your particular illness, you may need to take a specific drug on a regular basis. You may do better to take your painkillers spread out during the day at a regular time, and not wait until the pain has become really bad. Some people may successfully use painkillers more intermittently. It can make managing pain on a day-to-day basis easier if you know that you could choose to have a 'holiday' from pain from time to time. Almost anything is easier to cope with if you know that you could have moments when you could chose not to have to cope.

It can be worth thinking about how much help you are getting from your painkillers. If they are causing a lot of side effects, you might consider whether taking less of them might be better. Always discuss this with your doctor before cutting back.

Long-term use of painkillers can sometimes cause headaches. If you have headaches, do discuss this with your doctor.

Types of painkillers

There are many different kinds of analgesic drugs, some of which may be appropriate for your kind of pain. In this book, we are talking about long-term illness in general, rather than any one specific illness, so we cannot make recommendations abut any one analgesic. Even though some can be bought without a prescription, it is always worth talking to your doctor or specialist about what would be suitable for you and the best way to take it to reduce side effects. The more potent painkillers need to be prescribed by a doctor anyway. All we can do here is to give a summary of the different types.

Aspirin

This is readily available without prescription and may give relief. The disadvantage is that it can have the side effect of gastric problems if used a lot. Do not take it on an empty stomach.

Paracetamol (not available in the USA)

Again, this can be bought over the counter and can be helpful. If used at the recommended dose it is not dangerous.

Non-steroidal anti-inflammatory drugs (NSAIDS)

Drugs such as ibuprofen (Brufen or Neurofen) can sometimes help with pain in joints or muscles. They can cause stomach problems such as acid indigestion, though some of the latest versions may cause less. Ibuprofen is available without prescription, but other anti-inflammatory drugs may need one. Always take them with or after food. You may be prescribed additional drugs to help protect your stomach.

Antidepressants

A low dose of one of the antidepressant drugs such as amitryptiline (Tryptizol or Elavil) or Venaflaxine used on a regular basis can help with pain (whether or not you are depressed). They are often used in Pain Management Clinics for a variety of conditions causing pain. The dose is much lower than that used in treating depression, so they are not likely to have much in the way of side effects. They are not addictive in the sense of people needing more and more or being unable to stop taking them (although some people do report worsening of symptoms when they stop taking these drugs).

Codeine and opiates

These range in potency from those for moderate pain, e.g. codeine, to those for severe pain, e.g. morphine. Your pain may be severe enough to require the use of such drugs, but they do have side effects. They can cause severe constipation and interfere with sleep. They may also be addictive. As they have to be prescribed by a doctor, you will have a chance to discuss the best ways and time for taking them.

Combination drugs

There are several painkillers that contain two drugs, such as a combination of paracetamol and codeine. Though they can be effective, they have the drawback of reducing the scope for increasing or reducing just one of the drugs. You might be better off taking the two drugs separately.

Anti-convulsants

These drugs such as gabapentin (Neurontin) and carbamazepine (Tegretol), originally used for epilepsy, are being increasingly used to treat neuropathic pain. They may have side effects, but these can be minimized by starting at a very low dose and gradually increasing it.

Cannabis

We are aware that many people do use cannabis to help with their pain, even though it can be illegal. Research is being carried out to try to find a painkilling drug based on the active ingredients of cannabis, so at some time there may be drugs that a doctor could prescribe.

Another approach

If you are concentrating on reducing your pain, or not making it worse, you may tend to avoid any activity that you fear will produce pain. Paradoxically, this can make things worse by focusing your mind on pain and by limiting what you can do and enjoy. It might therefore be better to work on simply accepting some degree of pain, and focusing on enjoying what you do. If you can achieve this, at least for some of the time, you may well find that you have an improved quality of life, notice your pain less and have fewer of the unpleasant emotions associated with pain.

Further information

Coping Successfully with Pain, Neville Shone—a good self-help book.

Bandolier's Little Book of Pain—an evidence-based guide to treatments for pain.

Coping with Pain—a well balanced, informative cassette.

Coping with Chronic Pain—a very good, informative CD, which looks at ways you can help yourself both physically and emotionally. It finishes with a good section on relaxation.

Full Catastrophe Living, Jon Kabut-Zinn—How to cope with stress, pain and illness using mindfulness meditation.

10 Using activity and exercise

You may feel that, because of your illness, exercise is just not possible. Well, our message is that the *right* kind of exercise will help anybody, with whatever condition! Even if you are completely bedridden, passive exercise with someone else moving your limbs for you would be a help. Appropriate exercise is the key phrase. You may need to get expert advice to discover just what is right for you, but keeping your body in the best condition possible in the circumstances really is a good idea.

Are you suffering from the effects of inactivity?

You may have found that doing nothing for a day or two reduces some of your symptoms and so believe that more rest is the answer. However, though we all need reasonable periods of good quality rest, too much of it does not help our bodies. It can lead to muscle weakness, stiff joints, poor circulation and back problems. It also causes loss of motivation and poor concentration. Research for the American space programme has shown that prolonged rest—even for periods as short as 2 weeks—can cause such changes, even in fit young people.

Some of the problems and symptoms you are experiencing could be because you have got out of condition since you became ill. For instance, spending a lot of time lying in bed can make you feel weak and worsen back pain. Bodies are built to move. It will help your body if you can keep it moving, even if all you can manage is a small amount at intervals during the day. Little and often works well. Try to build appropriate periods of physical activity into your self-management plan. If you are uncertain where to start, you could ask for a fitness assessment from a physiotherapist, who would be able to plan out an exercise programme appropriate for the way you are now, or you might get advice from the specialist clinic that you attend.

Getting fitter

Try not to be over-ambitious. Forget what you used to do before you got ill. Just concentrate on what suits your body now, and work out what you can do comfortably and for how long. Warm up with gentle stretches and stop when you have completed what you planned. Do *not* carry on until you feel too tired to continue. A small amount done regularly is going to do you much more good than doing too much one day and then being too tired to do anything the next day. If you can find a type of exercise that you enjoy, you are much more likely to be able to keep it going.

Here are some suggestions about how you can help yourself:

- *Bending and stretching exercises*—joints that are not used get stiff like rusty hinges, muscles that are not used get shorter and weaker, so gentle exercises will help avoid problems. Start very gradually. You can do gentle exercises even while lying down. It is sometimes easier to do such exercises in warm water. If there is a swimming pool within easy reach, you could try using the learner pool (which is often at a higher temperature) at a quiet time.

- *Walking*—this is one of the best forms of exercise, even if you can only manage a small amount. Two short walks morning and afternoon are better than one longer one that leaves you exhausted. You will probably find that by splitting your walks into smaller chunks you will be able to walk further in total. Perhaps you may only be able to manage a few paces at first, but even that will be a good start. Walking briskly is very good for you, if you can manage it. Walking upstairs sometimes instead of using an elevator can be very good exercise.

- *Swimming and cycling*—if your condition allows it, these are both good forms of exercise if done gently and in moderation. Pace yourself carefully, always stopping before you get too tired.

- *Posture*—if you are feeling very tired or unwell, it is very tempting to slouch or sit in a slumped position. This is not going to help your body. Walking well (think tall!) will help. Equally, choosing the right kind of chair that allows you to sit in a good position is important. Both of these can reduce some pain.

- *Exercise classes*—depending on your particular illness, there may be exercise classes suitable for your condition. You might find it easier to have an instructor to guide you, and you might enjoy the social contact and the encouragement of participating in a group activity. For instance, many people suffering from arthritis have found specialized classes very helpful. Gentle yoga classes might be appropriate.

Alexander technique classes could help you improve your posture. Pilates' classes can improve core muscle tone. Some swimming pools run water aerobics classes, which can be helpful if you need to keep weight off your joints. Find out what is available locally, whether through your specialist clinic or in the community.

• *Pelvic floor exercises*—these are important for men as well as women. Keeping these up regularly will avoid a lot of problems later.

Benefits of exercise

There are so many different kinds of long-term illness that it is difficult to be specific about each and every one, but there are some generalities that we can point out.

Improvement in general health

The right kind and amount of exercise for you and your condition will certainly help your general health and be good for your heart and lungs. This will be of benefit as you grow older. Exercise will help to keep your body in the best condition possible and perhaps avoid other problems such as back pain or raised blood pressure. It could be part of your strategy for keeping your weight under control.

Stronger muscles

Stronger muscles will make life easier for you. If, for instance, you suffer from osteoarthritis, strengthening the muscles round an affected joint could reduce the pressures on that joint.

Improved joint mobility

Stiff joints would only add to your general problems. They can certainly add to pain.

Less pain

There have been many studies into long-term pain that show the benefits of exercise.

Possible slow-down in degeneration

Depending on your particular illness, appropriate exercise may make a potential degeneration happen at a slower rate. Again, taking osteoarthritis as an example, improved muscle tone may delay the need for a joint replacement or the need to have such a replacement revised.

Pleasure

Some people really enjoy exercise and get satisfaction from taking it. There is some evidence that exercise can release endorphins—chemicals in the brain that have painkilling properties and which give a sense of pleasure. Exercise can be a help if you are feeling depressed. Getting a little fitter will probably mean that you could do more of the things you enjoy and that would improve your quality of life.

Fears about exercise

It is all too common for people with a long-term illness to have cut back on physical activity for fear of making themselves worse. Equally, people who suffer from a painful condition may be afraid that doing something that hurts means that they are doing themselves harm. That is where expert advice can be so helpful. Having expert supervision of your exercise, at least at the beginning, can be very reassuring. You can be taught what movements will be beneficial and which to avoid.

Vanity

Do not discount the beneficial effects of vanity! It can be a real incentive to do some exercise. If you are walking better or have tightened up some slack muscles, you will certainly look better. This could be a boost to your self-esteem.

11 Improving your sleep

Most of us delight in 'a good night's sleep'. Unfortunately, sleep problems are common in many long-term illnesses and can add to fatigue and general misery. You may find it difficult to get to sleep, or you may wake often during the night. Sometimes, even if you have slept, you may still wake up feeling tired. These problems can increase fatigue and add to the general misery of illness, so it is worth looking at all the ways in which you could improve the situation.

Talk it over with your doctor

There are many causes of sleep problems, many of which are treatable. These can be the effects of some medications, stress, worry and depression. Bladder problems that mean getting up frequently to go to the toilet can disrupt sleep patterns. Pain can also disrupt sleep. See if your doctor can help in any way.

Getting to sleep

You can experiment with all the things that help you get to sleep, such as establishing a calm routine that leads up to bedtime, and relaxing when you get there. Try to avoid too much stimulation just before you go to bed—watching that exciting television programme, or reading a thriller could be a mistake. The period just before sleep is *not* the time for thinking about problems—which will make it much harder for you to settle down. Many people find it helpful to set up a specific 'worry time' earlier in the day. If you find yourself anxious about some problem while you are trying to get to sleep, tell yourself that you will think about it tomorrow during your worry time. Avoid alcohol and caffeine-containing drinks in the couple of hours before bed time—they may make it harder to get to sleep. A milky drink at bed time may help.

Is your bed really comfortable? If your mattress is old and not as comfortable as it used to be, you may need to think about replacing it. You could try experimenting with different arrangements of your pillows if you have problems with your neck. Is the temperature right for you—not too hot or not too cold? Anything that makes your bedroom an oasis of calm and peace will help. If you can, keep your bedroom for sleeping, rather than for other activities. If you find noise disruptive, such as a partner snoring, you could experiment with soft ear plugs.

Waking in the night

Try to stay calm and relaxed if you do wake. Build up a collection of gentle, pleasant things to occupy your mind. That way, you will still be getting rest and you are more likely to fall asleep again. Use your relaxation routine, which is likely to help you get back to sleep, but which will also give you the best quality rest while you are awake.

Worrying about not sleeping is almost guaranteed to keep you awake. It is only too easy to get caught up in thoughts like 'If I don't get back to sleep, I'll be hopeless in the morning. I won't be able to cope.' That is not necessarily so.

If you really cannot get back to sleep, get up, move to another room and occupy yourself with something gentle for a while such as reading or listening to music until you feel sleepy again. Talking books, particularly if the subject matter is not exciting and the reader has a calm voice, can be very helpful.

Pain and sleep

If pain is what makes it difficult to get to sleep, or what wakes you in the night, it is worth experimenting with all the things that help a little. Would it help if you changed the times at which you take your pain medication? Does a hot-water bottle placed against the sore area help? Could you keep an electric kettle in your bedroom so that you do not have to go to the kitchen to fill a hot-water bottle? Getting really relaxed and then distracting your mind from the pain by thinking about something pleasant and interesting may help too.

Establishing a regular pattern

You need to establish regular times for going to bed and for waking. Research has shown how important it is to keep the body's rhythms in a regular pattern. The effects of 'jet lag' show what happens when these are disrupted.

You may need to re-establish such a regular pattern to avoid sleeping at other times. If you have slept badly during the night, it is very tempting to sleep longer in the morning, but this is not always a good idea. An alarm clock or a timed radio can help you wake at a regular time. You can always rest later in the day if you need to. If you are feeling very tired, it may seem reasonable to have naps during the day. This may be the right thing for you, but it might make it more difficult to get to sleep at night. If you want a daytime nap and if it will fit into your schedule, try to have it at a regular time (like a 'siesta' after lunch). You can experiment to see what works best for you.

Using sedatives

If these simple 'sleep hygiene' methods are not enough, you might want to consider taking one of the several types of sedative medicine in consultation with your doctor.

Some kinds of antihistamines such as promethazine (Phenergan) or cyproheptadine (Periactin) have a sedating effect, and may be enough to help you sleep. They can be bought at a chemist without a prescription.

Another good alternative is to take a low dose of a sedative 'antidepressant' drug such as amitriptyline (Tryptizol or Elavil) or trazadone (Molipaxin or Desyrel) an hour or two before you go to bed. Such drugs are not just prescribed to help mood; they have a lot of useful effects for improving sleep and helping with pain. At this low dosage, they are very unlikely to have any unpleasant side effects. They are not addictive.

The most commonly prescribed sedatives are benzodiazepines such as Temazepam. They are safe and effective, but they can interfere with the quality of sleep. It is better to avoid using sleeping pills on a regular basis because you may become dependent on them (unlike antidepressants). They may make you sleep longer, but it will not be very good quality sleep. However, you could talk to your doctor about using them in a limited way. You may find it very much easier to deal with sleep problems if you know that you could give yourself an occasional 'holiday' from insomnia. If you are fretting about being awake a lot one night, you could reassure yourself by thinking 'Tomorrow night I could take a pill and sleep through the night'. It is much easier to cope with anything if you know you do not have to do it for ever.

12 Managing bladder and/or bowel problems

These can be very common for a lot of people, and can add to the difficulties of managing a long-term illness. If you suffer from them, it is always worth getting medical help and advice. Being afraid to go too far away from the toilet is very restricting and reduces your quality of life.

Bladder problems

Leakage from the bladder is all too common, especially in women, and usually occurs when you laugh, sneeze or exercise (stress incontinence). Other problems are:

- Often needing to hurry to the toilet to empty your bladder
- Needing to empty your bladder very many times a day
- Having to get up several times a night to go to the toilet
- Wetting the bed in your sleep—this can happen to people of all ages, not only children
- Your bladder does not empty completely
- You need adaptations to your home or your clothes to make going to the toilet easier
- You have memory problems that affect your ability to use the toilet.

The most important thing is that treatments are available for all these problems. Some people can be completely cured; others will feel a whole lot better. You might benefit from adaptations to your home or to your clothes to make going to the toilet easier. Expert advice is available from specialized clinics staffed by really helpful trained professionals.

Some people believe that these problems are inevitable as we grow older. That is not true. Others feel too embarrassed to talk about it. Do try to believe that though you may feel embarrassed, the health professionals you talk to will not. They will just think of it as something that they often meet and which they can do something about. Do your best to overcome your reluctance and talk to your doctor, a specialist continence advisor or a nurse.

One of the best ways to overcome minor leakages is to do pelvic floor exercises regularly. This applies to men as well as to women. It may take a few months for this to make a significant difference, but it will do if you persevere. Your doctor or a nurse can advise you on how to do these exercises.

We know that some people try to manage their problems by restricting their fluid intake. This is a serious mistake. In time, it just makes the bladder shrink and concentrates the urine, which can lead to bladder infections.

Bowel problems

Leakage from the bowel is much less common but even more distressing. Strengthening the pelvic floor muscles may help. There are also other techniques that your doctor can advise you about.

Other problems can include constipation or diarrhoea (or an alternation between the two states). Again, you should seek medical advice for these.

Further information

www.continence-foundation.org.uk. This site gives very helpful information and advice. You can also use it to find a local continence clinic. There are similar organizations in Canada and Australia.

13 Looking after your general health

If you have to manage a particular illness, looking after your general health becomes even more important. You need to do as much as you can not to burden your body with other problems. Long-term illness may well mean lifetime illness. As we get older, our chances of developing other problems increases, but the risk can be minimized by healthy living. Much of what we talk about in this book is about general health management as much as about illness management. So here is a summary of health behaviours that would be good sense for anybody, sick or well. You will find most of the following topics expanded on throughout the book.

Healthy eating

Good food is essential for health. There is good evidence that eating the right foods in the right amounts can reduce the risk of certain cancers and of getting heart disease. Eat at least five portions of vegetables and fruit every day, whole grain food at least four times a week and fish (including oily fish) twice a week. If you take a multivitamin tablet every day, make sure that it includes at least 200 micrograms of folic acid. Stick to a reasonably low fat, low sugar diet. There is more about a good diet in Chapter 14.

Weight control

Try to avoid gaining weight. It is very much easier to keep weight stable than to have to lose weight. If you do need to shed some pounds, do it slowly. Crash diets do not work in the long term. Reduce your calorie intake (and increase your exercise if that is possible) enough to lose no more than one pound a week. You may feel that doing it that way would take far too long to achieve your ideal weight, but in 3 months you could lose nearly 14 pounds. Once you have reached your target, try to keep to a diet with which you can keep your weight stable.

Exercise

Exercise will help to keep your body in good shape. If your condition allows it, try to do the kind of exercise that leaves you feeling a little breathless at least three times a week. This will be good for your heart and lungs. Regular exercise will strengthen bones, keep them strong and reduce the risk of osteoporosis. Doing the kind of exercise that keeps your back muscles strong and your joints mobile will help to reduce problems.

Stop smoking

If you can stop smoking, do it. Give all the suggested techniques a good try and, most importantly, make up your mind to stop. If you do carry on smoking, reduce your cigarettes to no more than five a day, and leave long portions of the day when you do not smoke.

Look after your teeth

If you are ill, the last thing you need is trouble with your teeth, so meticulous tooth care is worth the effort. Careful brushing (an electric toothbrush can make it easier if you are feeling frail) and the use of dental floss will help avoid trouble. At the very least, use a fluoride mouth rinse. Try to get regular check ups by your dentist if at all possible. You may be able to get a home visit by a dentist if you are really too ill to visit a dental surgery.

Look after your feet

There are some illnesses such as diabetes in which scrupulous foot care is vital, but it is a good idea for any one with a long-term illness. Your doctor may be able to refer you to a chiropodist (podiatrist), or you may be able to afford to visit one privately. There is a lot you can do for yourself. Keep your toenails cut regularly (get someone else to do it for you if you have difficulty reaching them yourself). Dry between your toes carefully. Wear the right, well fitting shoes so that you avoid problems such as blisters or bunions.

Sensible precautions

Discuss with your doctor the possibility of having an annual check-up during which you have some basic tests for such things as diabetes, high blood pressure or raised cholesterol. Such conditions are much better caught early and treated early.

Women should take advantage of offered cervical smear tests and mammograms. Ask your doctor to show you how to examine your breasts and then do so once a month.

Men should do self-checks on their prostate and testes. Again, ask your doctor if you are uncertain how to do it.

Further information

www.ebandolier.org.uk has useful information about sensible health behaviours.

14 Eating well and wisely

Good food, and the pleasure and nourishment you can get from it, should be part of your self-management plan. If you are feeling unwell or tired, it can be all too easy to neglect yourself, going for the easiest options in meals and eating at odd hours, but a good, varied diet is important for health. Maintain or get back into the habit of having meals at consistent, normal times—breakfast, lunch and supper. Some people feel better if they do not go too long between meals. If you are one of them, then including small, healthy snacks between meals can be a good idea.

A normal healthy diet

The following are generally accepted as part of a healthy diet: complex carbohydrates (wholemeal bread rather than white); pulses (beans, lentils, etc.); plenty of fresh fruit, salads and lightly cooked vegetables; good quality low-fat protein; milk and cheeses; eggs; liver (but not if you are pregnant); and oily fish (such as tuna and mackerel).

Try to include as much variety as you can in your meal planning. Eating healthily is important, but there is nothing wrong with the occasional bit of self-indulgence. For instance, eating a lot of chocolate would not be good for you, but having a small bar sometimes (particularly as a reward for good management) can be a lift to the spirits.

Food supplements

Your aim should be to get all the nourishment you need from what you are eating. You may be advised by some alternative therapists, or you may read on the Internet, that you should be taking a lot of supplements of vitamins and minerals to help manage your particular condition. There is very little evidence that this is necessary. Supplements like this can be very expensive. Nourishment is probably more easily absorbed from food than from pills.

It can be dangerous to take too much of some vitamins (such as vitamin A) and for others our bodies simply excrete what they do not need, so you could end up with most of what you have paid for disappearing down the toilet.

There may be times when your doctor suggests you need to supplement one particular vitamin or mineral. For instance, if you are at risk of osteoporosis because of a sedentary life style, then added calcium would be helpful. A multivitamin, multimineral pill once a day will not do you any harm and may do some good. Select one that contains folic acid.

Special diets

Some medical conditions, for instance coeliac disease, diabetes or renal failure, do require special diets. You need to get as much expert advice as you can. Your doctor or your specialist clinic will be able to help you. Other sources of information could be the support groups for your particular condition, who may publish information leaflets. The major supermarket groups can often be helpful too in supplying help and information. Sticking to your diet is very important, so the more sound advice you can get, with suggested dishes and cookery tips, the easier it will be for you and the better for your body. You could ask to be referred to a dietician.

Food allergy and sensitivity/intolerance

Some people blame their illness on what they eat. Some aspects of diet can lead to diseases. More often, people feel that they are allergic to certain foods. In fact, this is only rarely because of a true allergy, and allergy is a relatively uncommon way in which food can cause illness. An example is that some people are allergic to certain foods such as peanuts. If you do get definite symptoms of allergy—such as tingling and swelling of the tongue and lips, wheezing or rash—this is a potentially life-threatening problem. You must avoid that food and you should see your doctor.

More commonly, food is blamed for symptoms such as tiredness. If this is the case, even though you are not truly allergic to some foods, you may feel better if you exclude them from your diet. Some people do seem to be intolerant of gluten in their diet, even though they do not meet the criteria for true coeliac disease. Do be careful though—excluding too many foods may put your nutrition at risk and can certainly reduce your quality of life. If you do cut out a food, you need to think about replacing it with something else. For instance, if you cut out milk and milk products, you would need to find alternative sources of calcium such as calcium tablets, soy products and bony fish such as sardines.

Weight change

Being either overweight or underweight can be a problem. If you are taking much less exercise because of your illness and yet are still eating the same amount as you did before you became ill, it is very easy to put on weight. Comfort eating can also lead to weight gain. Carrying too much weight will only add to your fatigue and may lead to other health problems. Similarly, it is not helpful to lose too much weight. If you have a problem with your weight, talk to your doctor or to a dietician and get advice on a diet that will keep your weight stable.

Depression can produce problems of both weight loss and weight gain. Some people who are suffering from depression lose their appetite. Some of the drugs that are used to treat depression can have a side effect of increasing appetite and weight; others reduce them (see Chapter 22). Discuss this with your doctor if he or she is prescribing an antidepressant for you.

Tired of cooking (or tired by cooking)

Eating well does not mean that you have to spend a lot of time cooking. You can get all the nourishment you need from very simple food. For instance, a sandwich made from wholemeal bread, cold meat or tinned tuna, with a tomato or some fresh fruit, and a glass of milk is a perfectly healthy meal. If you choose to avoid certain foods such as wheat or milk products, then you would need to find simple alternatives.

You may find that there are certain times of day when you feel more like cooking. Planning ahead and doing food preparation in advance may save you from feeling too tired to tackle the job just before a meal. If you can afford them, a freezer and a microwave cooker can be very useful pieces of equipment, enabling you to cook on days when you feel up to it, and then to heat up something from the freezer on days when you really do not. Perhaps you could get a relative or a friend to do some cooking for you, to be stored in a similar way.

These days, there is a wide variety of ready meals available. Some of them can be very good, but some may have a high fat and salt content. Do check the labels. However, a few of them in the freezer could be a useful standby for days when you do not feel like cooking.

Keeping diet and food as normal as possible

One general rule that applies here is that it is better to do things as normally as possible unless there is a good reason not to. You may have received strong medical advice about a change of diet, which you do need to heed, but this can still be applied in a 'normal' way. You may realize that your previous eating habits included a lot of junk food and eating at irregular hours. If so, this is a good time to change to a regular, healthy diet, which would be something of benefit to you for the rest of your life.

Enjoying what you eat is one of the basic pleasures of life, so try to eat healthily and happily.

section 3
Managing emotional issues

15   Setting goals for yourself

Setting a goal for yourself and then achieving it can be a very satisfying experience. It is something we all do to a greater or lesser extent, and it can be a good way of improving your quality of life within a long-term illness. You are probably doing some of this already, but there may be things that you would like to accomplish, but have set aside because your illness seems to make them difficult. Difficult, however, does not mean impossible. Done in a different way or at a slower pace, some of your goals might be attainable. You may feel that your life would be more satisfying if you could do more physically or mentally, or if you could do more with other people. All this could be part of your self-management plan. You will already have your own way of thinking about what you want to achieve, but may find the following structured approach useful. It looks at both picking out a goal and working out what would need doing to achieve it.

Choosing a goal

Think about all the things you would like to do or which you think would be helpful (not always the same thing!) You may have been told by your doctor that you should be taking more exercise, or doing your best to lose some weight. Such recommendations could be included in your list of goals. It can help if you write out your list, being careful to keep each item separate and clear. Then you can choose just one of them—something you want to do or achieve in the foreseeable future, which you feel is within your power. You can then check whether it is an appropriate goal by considering some of the following points and questions (depending on your goal, not all of them will be relevant):

- Write down your goal in a very specific way. Is it realistic? Re-write it if necessary.
- What would be the benefit to you if you did achieve it? What might be the benefits for anyone else?

that, she will slowly increase the distance she walks, being careful not to be too ambitious.

By the end of 6 weeks, she has managed to get to the park and is feeling very proud of herself. She enjoyed chatting to her neighbour who walked with her for the first couple of weeks and is now confident that she can keep going on her own. She has met a couple of nice women in the park who walk their dogs there. From now on, she makes a point of walking at least 3 days a week. Her husband is really pleased and they are making plans for little expeditions that they can take together. As a reward, she buys herself a nice pair of new shoes.

Another method

An alternative approach may also suit you. This is to imagine as strongly as you can the new development you want. After you have chosen your goal and have checked whether this is realistic, concentrate on all the details of how this would feel. This is very similar to the way that top athletes visualize themselves running at their fastest, or making the perfect tennis stroke. Concentrating on all the details of what this would be like and how they would feel really does improve their performance. This can be the same for you.

16 Dealing with problems

Coping with difficulties and problems is a part of normal life. However, being ill can create a new batch of problems to add to the ones you had before. At every stage of your illness, things change; some things that are difficult get easier, but new difficulties crop up. We all have our own ways of coping, but the problems generated by illness will make new demands on your ability to cope and may require some 'advanced coping skills' (another term for dealing with problems). Managing problems in the best way is very much part of managing your illness and making life easier for yourself.

Before going on to consider how best to cope with problems, you might like to think about the difference between difficult circumstances and soluble problems. Many of the people we talk to seem to be trying to solve the difficult circumstances rather than the problems caused by these circumstances. To give an example, it is raining and you are afraid of getting wet if you go out. The rain is the circumstance, about which you can do nothing. The problem is getting wet, which you can tackle by using an umbrella or wearing a rain coat.

Do keep in mind that some problems do not have obvious solutions. Part of your technique for dealing with problems should be to accept that some things may have to be tolerated for the time being. You may also have to accept that you may have to postpone addressing some problems until you have gathered more information. You cannot make realistic decisions until you know enough about your options.

When you are feeling ill and tired, problems tend to loom larger. It is very likely that you will have times when your problems feel overwhelming. It can then be hard to know where to start and how to find any solutions. If you can separate out your problems and deal with them one by one, your feeling of being overwhelmed will diminish. Your first step therefore is to define and list your separate problems. With each problem that you solve, you will get better at dealing with others and you will build up confidence in your own abilities.

It is worthwhile thinking back to a problem you tackled successfully in the past. How did you define what that problem was? How did you find a solution that worked? If a particular style of dealing with problems really works for you, then you can try it again. However, it could still be worth your while to read the next bit and then consider whether you could add the techniques we recommend to what you already do.

Problem solving

One of the life skills that will be particularly useful to you now is called 'problem solving'. There has been a lot of research that has looked at the best way of dealing with problems. What follows is just a summary of the technique. Work through it and then, if you find it useful, you can see more detail in a book we recommend at the end of this chapter.

What we suggest is that you start with just one fairly simple problem. Choose one that you know could be solved. You can then tackle it in seven stages.

Stage 1: identifying and clarifying the problems

It is going to be much easier to tackle problems if you can identify exactly what they are and separate out each one from all the other stuff that is bothering you. Make a written list of them all, thinking very carefully about exactly what each one is and how important it is to you. It may help if you ask yourself the following questions:

- What exactly is the problem? (Tip—be as realistic as you can about it.)
- How does it make you feel?
- When and where does the problem occur?
- What other people does it involve?

Be very specific; do not muddle this problem up with others. Give it a name. Write down a clear description of the problem and be sure to make the problem very precise. Sometimes people choose too large a problem which can be difficult to tackle. If the problem seems too large, try chopping it into smaller bits and tackle only a small bit of the problem at a time. An analogy is called 'breaking the bundle' like trying to break a bundle of twigs. It may be impossible to break the whole bundle, but quite easy to break the twigs one at a time.

Jenny has had breast cancer, which seems to have been successfully treated by surgery and chemotherapy. However, the treatment has left her experiencing extreme fatigue. One of the many problems this causes is that she is often too tired to feel like cooking a meal and so just eats snacks. As a result, she has a very poor diet and is beginning to lose weight, which worries her and her doctors. The weight loss makes her afraid that the cancer has returned.

So she says that the problem is that she is not eating enough of the right food.

Stage 2: deciding on your goal or goals

Set yourself a goal of what would be better, rather than a somewhat vague hope for improvement. Choose a realistic goal that you know you can achieve and make it precise. You need to be able to state what the difference is that you are looking for.

Jenny decided that she wanted to get back to eating three good meals a day. Breakfast (of muesli and fruit) was not a problem, but she needed to find ways of achieving a good lunch and supper in spite of her fatigue. She hoped that she would then stop losing weight. That would make her feel better in body and mind.

So her goal is to eat a good lunch and supper.

Stage 3: thinking of as many solutions as possible

'Brainstorming' means thinking about as many solutions as possible— even ones that may seem silly initially—and is a useful technique. It is a good idea to use a pencil and paper at this stage. Your aim is to identify as many solutions as possible, writing them down, and not stopping to think about whether any of them would work until you have run out of ideas. Having someone you trust doing this with you can be useful as they might be able to suggest ideas that you might not have thought about. You do not need to reject *any* idea at this stage, even if it seems to be ridiculous. Do not stop and say 'Oh but that wouldn't work'. Only when you have got your complete list in front of you should you start to evaluate the solutions. Ask yourself what might be the advantages and disadvantages of each one.

Jenny decided to ask her friend Anna (who does her shopping for her) to help with the brainstorming. Together they brainstormed a list of solutions that included getting Meals on Wheels to bring her lunch, buying good quality ready prepared meals, phoning for take-away meals, paying someone to come in and cook for her every day, asking Social Services for help, Jenny cooking some simple casseroles in the morning (when she felt less tired) and freezing portions to eat on other days, getting the right ingredients to make healthy sandwiches to eat with fruit or salad, Anna coming in once a week to do a lot of cooking and then freezing single portions.

Stage 4: choosing the best solution and deciding how to put it into practice

When you have got your list of solutions in front of you, you can choose what seems to be the best solution. This is the one that seems to be the most achievable and which fits your situation best.

Jenny decided that she wanted to be as independent as possible, so she did not want to depend on Anna's help in cooking (though she was grateful for the offer), or have a helper from Social Services coming in. She preferred to choose what she ate rather than depending on Meals on Wheels. She could not afford to pay someone to cook for her or to buy ready prepared meals more than occasionally. She felt that she could do some cooking for herself (which she used to enjoy), if she did it at the right time of day and had the right ingredients and equipment.

When you feel happy about the solution, break it down into steps. 'I could start by doing this and then move onto doing that.' Be very definite about what you are going to do and when you are going to do it.

Jenny decided that her steps would be:

- To order an electric slow cooker (so that she could cook simple casseroles without having to check them while they were cooking) and a supply of plastic boxes, suitable for single portions, from a mail order catalogue.
- She and Anna would revise her shopping list to include cold meat and wholemeal bread to make healthy sandwiches for lunch, plenty of fruit and salad, and the ingredients for casseroles, as well as a few good quality ready meals to store in the freezer.
- She would prepare a casserole at least three times a week, which would give one portion to eat that day and one to put into the freezer in a plastic box.
- After breakfast, she would prepare sandwiches for lunch, which she would eat with fruit or salad.
- During the afternoon, she would prepare some vegetables to eat with supper.
- Early in the evening, she would put the vegetables on to cook and heat up a portion of a casserole in the microwave. Occasionally, if she was feeling especially tired, she would use one of the ready meals from the freezer, or order a take-away meal.

Stage 5: trying it out

There is no point in having a potential solution if you do not try it. If you start finding good reasons *not* to try out the solution, it was probably not the right one, or you may have chosen too big a problem to begin with and would perhaps do better to tackle just part of the problem.

Once Jenny got going, she found that she could cope with cooking in the morning, as well as the small amount of effort involved in making sandwiches and preparing vegetables during the afternoon. She began to enjoy her healthier diet and eating regular meals.

Stage 6: evaluating the success of the solution

When you have put the solution into practice, check on whether it is working. It can be helpful to discuss this with someone. You will have learned a lot from any mistakes you have made.

Though Jenny was pleased that she was now eating more healthily and had stopped losing weight, she began to feel that a diet of sandwiches and casseroles was a little boring. She thought that she could probably manage to make soup (which used to be one of her specialities) some mornings, which she could then have at lunchtime. She also decided that she could probably cope with some very simple cooking in the evening—a piece of fish cooked in the microwave, an omelette or a grilled chop. She and Anna adjusted the shopping list with this in mind. Now that her diet was so much better, Jenny's fatigue was not quite so bad and she had stopped losing weight. She began to look forward to the time when she could do more for herself, perhaps going shopping with Anna so that she could select what food she would like to buy.

Stage 7: reviewing progress and beginning again

If the problem is solved, congratulate yourself. If not, start again at step 1 and decide if it was the best problem to tackle or whether the problem was too big and needed 'chopping into smaller bits'. Some questions to ask yourself could be:

- Was the definition of the problem too vague?
- Was it too big? Do you need to break it into smaller parts?
- Was it too hard? Do you need to choose an easier one to start with?
- Did you give your solution a fair try?

If you still think it was the right one to start with, try an alternative solution and progress through the stages as last time. You can then go on to tackle other problems in the same way.

Further information

Manage Your Mind, Gillian Butler and Tony Hope—Chapter 8.

17 Building pleasure into your life

If you are feeling tired and ill, it can be hard to think about enjoying yourself. You may have a Puritanical feeling that you do not deserve pleasure while you are ill or you may feel that some people will criticize you for using some of your available energy on things other than the essentials. However, pleasure *is* an essential part of your life—just as important as good food. Sometimes the things that you used to enjoy are not possible at present, but that does not mean that you could not enjoy yourself in rather different ways. Now could be the time to try something a bit different or to use a bit of lateral thinking to see if you could continue to do something you enjoy, even if you have to tackle it in a rather different way.

Mary Anne has had a stroke, which has left her with restricted movement of her left hand. She had always got a lot of pleasure from her skilful embroidery and did not want to give it up. She found a stand that would hold the embroidery hoop. She got the carer who came in once a day to thread several needles with the coloured threads she wanted. Now she can do small amounts of embroidery using just her right hand.

You could try making a list of all the things you can think of that might give you pleasure or satisfaction, within the limits of your condition. Keep it by you and add to it every time a new idea occurs to you. You might be surprised by how long a list you end up with. Most people have things that they always wanted to do but never had the time to try. This could be the moment to do some of them.

Irene is housebound much of the time because of her chronic bronchitis. Her windows look out over a garden, so she can watch the birds which she enjoyed, though she did not know much about them. She decided to buy a pair of binoculars and an illustrated book on birds so that she could study them more carefully and learn more. She now gets a great deal of pleasure in identifying the birds that she sees, and has taken part in a project to list garden birds in her area.

If you like flowers, it could be a good idea to keep a small vase by your bed in which you regularly put just one flower. Looking at this and really seeing all its details could be just as valid a pleasure as walking all the way round a botanical garden.

This could be a time for you to learn about subjects that have always interested you. Education does not just have to be about vocational training; it can be satisfying in its own right. Going to a class could be a good way of meeting people with similar interests. If getting out is difficult, you may be able to study by post or on the Internet. If one of your symptoms is fatigue, you may well find that when you are very tired concentration and mental effort become more difficult. This is another good reason for pacing yourself carefully, so that you can enjoy the pleasures of intellectual activity.

Michael enjoys music and gets great pleasure from listening to opera. When he had to take early retirement because of Parkinson's disease, he decided that rather than just listening, he would study the libretti of his favourite operas. He found that it added a great deal to his enjoyment to understand all the words of the arias.

Many people with a long-term illness find that this is a time to explore their creative side—art, writing, and so on. You could try writing something, purely for your own enjoyment, or to express just how you feel about your illness. You might even discover that you have a talent for it, perhaps to the extent that you get something published, which would do a lot for your self-esteem.

I always envied the other members of my family who were successful writers, but thought that it was a talent that had passed me by. Getting our book on CFS/ME published meant a very great deal to me. Frankie

Even if you do not think that you are any good at art, just putting colours on paper can be very satisfying. You might enjoy the tactile pleasures of working with clay. Experiment with different mediums and find out what gives you pleasure.

If you do not already have a pet, have you considered having one now? A dog which needs a lot of exercise might not be the most suitable, but perhaps you would enjoy having a cat. Stroking fur is said to help reduce stress. A tank of fish could give you something interesting to watch. A budgerigar does not require very much care, but can be fun. What do you think you might like?

You know best what you might enjoy. Experiment, always remembering that fun is possible and that it will do you a lot of good. You really do have the right to enjoy yourself and indulge yourself.

Treats and rewards

One way of looking at things could be to imagine what you would do for friends in similar circumstances. You might buy flowers for them, pick out an amusing book, choose a nice video or get some food that you know they enjoy. Have you considered indulging yourself in this way? Why not give yourself these sorts of little treats, if only as a reward for the way you are coping with your illness.

Keeping in contact with the outside world

Unfortunately, being ill can sometimes mean that you lose out on a lot of the social activity you enjoyed before. Feeling isolated can be a very common problem in illness. Social contact is a basic human need and very necessary for you now. You may have to think about being social in a rather different way, such as having a friend join you for a take-away meal instead of inviting several people round for a meal you prepared yourself. You may need to structure your social contacts for shorter periods than you used to enjoy.

You may also need to replace the friends who dropped away because they could not cope with you being ill (your illness may have reminded them of their own potential vulnerability). Making new contacts can often seem difficult, but usually there are ways round the problem. There may be a support group for your particular condition in your area that you could join and meet people with similar problems. If you cannot get out easily, there may be local organizations that do home visits (perhaps one of the churches near you). Maybe you could use problem solving to give you different ideas.

Socializing does not have to happen face-to-face. Pen-friends (a post-card, even if you cannot manage a letter) and telephone contacts can be very helpful. You could see if you could find compatible spirits through an Internet chat room dedicated to your condition or to your own special interests. E-mails can be a good way to keep in touch with friends. Anything you can do to keep in contact with the world is going to be good for you and lift your spirits.

Enriching your inner life

If your external life has been diminished by illness, then working on enriching and expanding your inner life could be important. How could that be done? Could you find ways of giving yourself more interesting things to think about? The poet who wrote 'my mind to me a kingdom is' was making a good point. Perhaps you could study something that has always interested you and extend your knowledge of it. Could you explore different kinds of music? Listening to the radio or watching television in a structured way can be helpful. You could try looking through the published list of programmes and marking up interesting things that you might like to listen to or watch.

Many people with a long-term illness feel that a spiritual dimension to their lives is very important to them. Some of them have a strong religious faith, but it is possible to experience spirituality without this. One definition of spirituality is 'looking inwards to discover our true identity' The 'looking inwards' is discovering who we are, what are our values and what gives meaning and purpose to our lives. Our 'true identity' is our essence and some would say it is experienced as peaceful and is expressed as compassion. Spirituality can also be thought of as a journey, a journey of self-discovery, which leads not only inwards but ultimately outward to the realization of the connection we have with all human beings and an experience of something greater than ourselves.

This could be something that you might wish to explore. It might add mental richness to a life which feels physically diminished by illness.

18 Living with uncertainty

Nobody feels comfortable with uncertainty, though people vary in how well they can tolerate it. A very basic human need is to feel certain about our life, which is actually an unobtainable goal—because life *is* uncertain. You cannot know for sure what is going to happen. Having a long-term illness adds to the areas of uncertainty. You may worry about whether a past decision was right or about what the future may hold.

The desire for a definitive disease diagnosis goes along with the need for some kind of certainty. If you have one of those illnesses that doctors have difficulty diagnosing or are reluctant to give a label to, it makes it so much harder to manage whatever you have. There may come a time though when you will have to accept that you are not going to get what you want and are going to have to settle for uncertainty. Better that than continuing with an ongoing search for a doctor who will be able to give you a label.

It is all too easy to spend a lot of time thinking about past decisions 'Should I have chosen that doctor or that treatment? 'Should I have asked more questions?' What if I had done such-and such?' 'It would have been so much better if I hadn't said such-and-such.' The fact remains that you did make those decisions. You may decide that you could now take further actions to rectify some past mistakes, but you cannot change the past. If you can now let it go, it would be much easier for you.

Uncertainty about the future is something different. The course of an illness can never be established totally. You might stay the same, get worse or even get better. Other things could crop up that might change the outcome. There is always the hope of a medical breakthrough that would change the prognosis of your particular illness. If you stay the same, at least you have a rough idea of how you can cope with it. Getting worse could bring a lot of new problems, though getting better can produce its own problems too. All sorts of other things might happen, over which you have very little control.

So what is it like living with uncertainty? Well, for a start, it is deeply uncomfortable. It can produce many other emotions and states of mind:

- Frustration—at your inability to achieve certainty.
- Anger—often directed at doctors for not being able to give you a definite answer.
- Vulnerability—not knowing what the future holds can leave you feeling vulnerable and anxious.
- Irritability—uncertainly can leave you feeling irritable with all those around you.
- Apprehension—you may have an uneasy feeling that the world is somehow dangerous.
- Fear—of possible futures, which is more difficult to manage as you cannot know for sure what they might be.
- Stubbornness—being very obstinate about some decisions.
- Possible loss of self-esteem.
- Exaggerated need for information—a constant search for the information to end the uncertainty.
- Blame—whether of yourself or other people.

Uncertainty can hold you back from making useful changes. You may not like the position you are in now, but feel hesitant about any change because you cannot be certain how it will turn out. Such 'safety first' thinking and behaviour can be very restricting.

One way that some people deal with uncertainty is to work towards getting the maximum control over some part of their lives—'If I can't control what goes on in the office, at least I'll keep my desk rigidly tidy.' That may seem to be comforting, but it really does not change anything much, and it may stop them finding better ways of dealing with it.

Learning to accept that you have only limited control over the future might be a better way. Managing the discomfort of uncertainty is probably the best option. Today is your only certainty, so dealing as well as you can with what is happening now will give you more confidence that you will deal reasonably well with whatever tomorrow might bring, uncertain though that may be.

19 Managing your thinking

Understanding the way you as an individual think about things—the way you view yourself, your life and the world around you—can make a great difference to the way you manage your illness. We all of us, well or ill, have our own established patterns in the way we think. Some of them are helpful and some unhelpful, but they all influence our thinking and our moods. Moods and emotions have a physical effect on the body, which is why we believe that managing your thinking is so important. Some of your beliefs and thought patterns may well have been appropriate in the past but no longer fit the person you are today.

We can point out some common ways of thinking and mention how they can get in the way of good management of an illness, but you are going to be the best person to judge just how much you think in these ways. We are *not* saying that the only reason you are ill is because of the way you think. What we *are* saying is that changing some unhelpful thought patterns may make life less difficult for you and make it easier for you to stick to your self-help programme.

Unhelpful thinking

Thinking that the worst is likely to happen

You may have got into the habit of always expecting the worst, of believing that if anything can go wrong for you then it will do. This can make things a lot more difficult for you if you are ill. You are likely to fear that any new symptom means that your illness is deteriorating or even that it is a sign of a life-threatening disease. If you expect things to turn out badly, you are likely to be hesitant at trying anything new.

Black and white thinking

In this style of thinking, everything is either good or bad, helpful or unhelpful, perfect or a disaster. If you stick to just black and white, you can miss out on the interesting shades of grey in between. You are likely to consider that you are either perfectly well or hopelessly ill, when the realistic viewpoint might be that you are not very well, but not as bad as you might be. Often events are seen as either successes or catastrophes, whereas in reality most are mixed—bits of good and bad. If you think this way, you are likely to believe that if you did not do something perfectly you failed, instead of thinking (accurately) that you did pretty well in the circumstances.

Negative thinking

This is very common, particularly if you are feeling a bit depressed. You are likely to always believe the worst, particularly about yourself and the way people are reacting to you. Typical thoughts could be:

- I'm a failure.
- I always get things wrong.
- Everybody dislikes me.
- I'll never be able to manage my illness.

If you look again at the last three thoughts, you will see that they contain very absolutist words such as 'always', 'everybody' and 'never'. This is very typical of negative thinking, when other words such as 'sometimes' and 'some people' would be much more accurate and 'never' could be replaced by a concept like 'it may take me some time'. Identifying and challenging these negative thoughts and looking at alternative, more accurate ones can make things look a lot better.

Mind reading

This is a very common problem. You presume that you know what people are thinking about you and it is usually rather negative. 'They think I'm not trying hard enough.' 'They don't believe that I'm really that ill.' That *might* be true, but it might not be. Checking up on the accuracy of your beliefs rather than jumping to conclusions is always worthwhile.

'Socially desirable' thinking

Another important area to consider is your own model of what makes you a 'good person'. In a society that is very much concerned with achievement, you may well feel devalued by being able to do much less. If you have had to give up your job, your own sense of worth may have sunk. The way of thinking you had before you were ill may have worked then, but may be totally inappropriate to your state now. It can be very helpful to look at your own ideas and judge whether they are helpful or unhelpful. The 'good person' way of thinking can often lead you to believing that you ought to be doing more than is appropriate or worrying that you are not doing enough. Our impression is that women tend to be more susceptible to pressures in this way, often believing that they ought to give their own needs a lower priority than those of their family or those around them.

Guilt

Another type of thinking that comes up a lot in long-term illness is guilt. So many of the people we talk with feel guilty about some aspect of their illness. This is often tied up with the concept of 'blame'. You may find it helpful to consider whether you would blame someone else in your position. If we suggest ways in which people could manage their illness better, we are certainly not blaming them for being ill. Some people tend to assume that if you become ill and stay ill, you are somehow at fault. A suggestion that you are just lazy can make things even worse. Such comments are ignorant and unfair and can make managing illness so much more difficult. Do your best to ignore them.

Doing something about unhelpful thinking

So what if you have decided that some of your thought patterns are unhelpful? What can you do about it? There are some well-tried and tested methods of challenging inappropriate and outdated thinking. Mostly they consist of asking yourself questions like:

- 'What is the evidence that supports this belief—is it really true?'
- 'Would I apply these standards to somebody else I cared about? Am I applying different standards to myself?'

You can get better at recognizing unhelpful thinking and then challenging it—along the lines of:

- 'OK, that is one way of thinking; that is one interpretation of events. Are there any others?'
- 'What could I do to find out whether this thought is accurate? Would it help if I discussed it with someone I trust?'

There is more about this in Chapter 23 and there are details in Appendix 2 of some books that you could find helpful.

Other things to consider

There are some other ways of thinking about yourself and your illness that can improve or diminish your well-being.

Aiming for normality

However severe your condition, there is more to your life than your illness. You are still a person of worth, even though you are ill, and you can contribute to life and take an interest in things other than illness. You do not have to think about yourself as *only* a person with your condition. The more you concentrate on your illness and the difficulties of your life now, the worse you are likely to feel—so do your best not to. Thinking and behaving in as normal a way as possible in the circumstances is going to make your life better. You need to balance sensible behaviour with the need to be 'ordinary'.

Balancing acceptance and hope

So many people with a long-term illness tell us that they can look back and see that real improvement in their life started only after they *accepted* what was happening to them. 'This is not what I wanted. I do not have to like it, but it is what is actually happening today. So how can I make the best of this situation?' This kind of acceptance does not mean that you have to give up hope for future improvement, rather the reverse. It is only when you are accurate in your thinking about today that you can start working on an improved tomorrow and so be more hopeful about the future.

20 Managing your self-esteem

Self-esteem means your personal feeling of self-worth. This is likely to be of great importance to your quality of life. You may have previously had good self-esteem, or you may perhaps have always had problems with this. Whichever is the case, a long-term illness can undermine your sense of self-worth in a variety of ways. It can change your whole idea of who you are and what makes you a valuable and valued person. You may have lost your good looks or physical prowess, the beautiful, active, healthy body you once had, and feel a loss of value because of that. Your illness may have caused a disfigurement. You may feel less effective as a parent, partner or carer. If you have had to give up your job, you may feel that you have lost your position as an achieving person. You may have lost some of your independence and now have to accept help from other people (and perhaps feel that you ought to be grateful, even though you hate having to ask for help).

If you are not now working, there can be other losses associated with giving up your job. Our society tends to value people for what they *do*, so if you have stopped *doing* in that sense you may feel you have lost esteem in the eyes of others. You may well have lost the companionship of the workplace and even feel as if you have become invisible.

Nevertheless, your achievements cannot be taken away from you. Now may be a time for using your abilities to address new challenges. One way to do this might be to do some voluntary work, even if it is only for an hour or two per week, which could give you a feeling of still being of worth.

Here are a few examples of people who have found new ways of making themselves feel valuable again. See if any of them could give you ideas for yourself:

JoAnn became paralysed from the waist down after a riding accident. She is now involved in a local campaign to improve facilities and access for the disabled.

Tom, who has MS, is still working, but has had to give up the sports he really enjoyed, particularly football. However, he has now started doing a little coaching for a local boys' soccer team.

Alice has rheumatoid arthritis and has had to give up her job as a reporter. She still writes the occasional article for newspapers and magazines, but has started working on writing fiction, beginning with short stories.

Jake has emphysema. He was the finance director of a large company. He used his financial expertise to investigate all the benefits to which he was entitled, and is now sharing what he has learnt with others in his self-help group.

Maryanne has heart disease. She took a course on watercolour painting and was delighted to have two of her pictures included in a local exhibition.

It is important to preserve and improve your sense of self-esteem. Here are some suggestions that may help.

Remember that you can still do and be. What you achieve and contribute may be different, but it could be just, or even more, worthwhile and valued. Your increased awareness of your own frailty may make you more understanding and accepting of others and deepen relationships with them.

Give yourself just credit for the way you are coping with your illness. Much of what you are achieving may not be obvious to other people, but you know what it is. Do your best not to think that someone else would do it much better.

Beware of making unhelpful comparisons. It is easy to compare yourself with other people, to help you to feel either good about yourself or bad about yourself. Mostly, if we are feeling bad about ourselves, we tend to assume that everyone else is doing better than we are. That is not necessarily so. It is all too easy to concentrate on the bits of other people's lives that seem admirable and forget the rest. In terms of developing your self-esteem, it is more helpful to see how you yourself are coping with your challenges. Be your own benchmark. Do your best to concentrate on what you *are* rather than what you *do*. Remind yourself that though you may not be able to *do* things for your children or family in the way you used to, you can *be* for them in a way that could be even more valuable. One of the ways in which you can still contribute is by being a role model in the way in which you cope with adversity.

Comparing yourself with what you did before you got ill is usually a mistake. There are new challenges now and new targets. Qualities and abilities you had before you became ill can still be useful, but the focus of these talents will be different. So be fair to yourself when you compare your present achievements with your own pre-illness standards.

Giving yourself proper credit for any achievement, no matter how small, is a good idea. Setting yourself small, realistic targets can help give you a valuable sense of achievement. Rate such achievement accurately. A small achievement may have taken a great deal of effort. You may tend to think that your illness stops you doing a lot of things that would give you satisfaction or a sense of achievement. That is not necessarily so. Having goals is important. (See 'Goal setting' in Chapter 15).

The way that you look does matter. It can help if you are able to continue or come back to taking pride in your appearance (at least some of the time). A becoming though easily maintained hairstyle, using make-up or shaving regularly, even if nobody else can see the results, or buying a new item of clothing (mail order can be useful) will all have a good effect on your morale.

It is very easy to concentrate on what goes wrong. Paying as much, or more, attention to what you are getting right can help to redress the balance. Thinking well of yourself is important. If you only look at what you are getting wrong, you are likely to have a lower opinion of yourself than if you pay equal attention to what you are getting right. One way to identify what works for you might be to keep a journal for a few weeks in which you only record successful events and good times. Once you can see what they were and how you achieved them, you can plan to do more in the same way.

Pay attention to how you are thinking about yourself. Catch yourself up if you realize that you are using unhelpful labels about the way you are or what you are able to do. If you call yourself a failure or pathetic, you just reinforce your lack of self-esteem. Be accurate about yourself. (See 'Talking to yourself' in Chapter 24).

Remember that your worth resides in what you are and not just in what you do. You can be able hearted, even though you are not able bodied. Concentrating more on the value of what you *are* than on what you *do* can be important now.

Further information

Overcoming Low Self-esteem, Melanie Fennell.

21 Managing your emotions

Managing the emotions and feelings that go with a long-term illness is as important as managing the physical problems. Mind and body cannot be separated. Emotions and moods have a physical effect on the body, and what happens to the body, and how you react to it, has an effect on the mind.

If you are ill, you are likely to have moments when you experience feelings of loss, envy, anger, frustration, worry and anxiety, fear or low spirits. You may find that stress makes you feel worse and that you do not cope with it as well as you once did. Old problems may still be with you, and you may notice them more now that you have less to distract you from them.

These emotions can be very powerful. However, there is much you can do to manage them, or to lessen the effect they have on you. Anything you can do to lift your spirits will be of value. It may help if you can find someone who feels able to listen when you need to talk about what is happening to you. Just putting things into words and hearing yourself telling your story can help. It is often more successful if the person you choose to confide in is not someone with whom you are emotionally involved—talking about these sorts of things to a partner or a close relative can get mixed up with aspects of your relationship and end up with both of you becoming distressed. If you do not have anyone whom you can confide in comfortably, then putting down your feelings on paper, or recording yourself talking about them can be surprisingly helpful. You may also benefit from seeking some expert help, particularly if you feel overwhelmed by your feelings.

If you have an illness that does not have a firm disease diagnosis, you may well be hesitant about admitting to having emotional problems, fearing that doctors or those around you will believe that your distress only proves that your illness is psychological after all. Even if you do find it hard to discuss such problems with most people, it will help if you can find someone safe to confide in. At least admit them to yourself.

We said earlier that what happens to the body has an effect on mood. For instance, you may well find that getting too tired can lower your spirits. If you are feeling particularly low, it is worth checking on your state of fatigue. It can be comforting to realize that this could be a transient misery—just a symptom—and that you will probably feel better after a good rest.

Improving your mood

Finding ways of improving your mood should be part of your self-help programme. This will both improve your quality of life and lessen the strain on your body. So let us look at some of the emotions you may be experiencing and think about what might help.

Loss and grief

Long-term illness almost always involves losses. These losses may cause grief. You may grieve for the person you used to be before you became ill, the body you used to have, the things that you once could do, maybe for the loss of a career and the companionship of the workplace. You may feel a sense of loss for the things you hoped to do which are now not possible.

One of the most painful losses can be having to give up the hope of having children, perhaps because the necessary treatment for your illness has caused infertility, or because you realize that you would not now be able to cope with pregnancy or with a child. Whilst there may not be anything you can do to change this reality, it may help how you feel if you can acknowledge and share these feelings.

Many of the people we have talked to mourn these losses almost as deeply as they would the death of a relative or a close friend. Talking about it will probably help a little, particularly if you can find someone to talk to who understands about bereavement.

> I certainly mourned the person I had lost by becoming ill. I went through all the emotions associated with bereavement, and could recognize them again when my husband died. Acknowledging the grief did help. The strength of feeling gradually eased, and though now I get a pang from time to time, it isn't the sharp grief I once experienced. Frankie

Although illness frequently involves losses, there may be some small gains as well. For instance, you may have had to give up a successful career, but find that you now have more time to enjoy your children. It helps if you can pay as much attention to any gains, however small, rather that just concentrating on your losses.

Envy

One of the things that can add to your emotional discomfort is an envy of other people who still have and can do the things you once had, could do or hoped to do. You would not be human if you did not envy people you know who are getting on with their lives, having a career, playing sports, marrying, having children, travelling, and those sort of things. Acceptance of your present condition is not easy. One thing that can help a little is to think about one particular person you envy. Instead of concentrating on the part of their life you wish you had, consider their whole package. Would you want all of it? Would you want her very difficult mother-in-law or his worry about being made redundant?

Frustration

It can be very frustrating not to be able to do the things that you used to do and enjoy, or to find yourself unable to take part in the life around you in the way you would like. It can be very tempting to think a lot about what is not possible and to get angry about it.

But what about the things you *can* still do? Are you giving them as much weight as what you cannot do? Could you do more of the possible sort of things? Building pleasure into today is really important. The more that you can improve your life now, the less energy you will spend on regretting the past. Come back into the present, leaving the past behind you, and explore what is possible now and how to get more of it. Sometimes, by changing the way in which you do things, you can achieve at least part of what you want. You could try making a list of all the things you still can do that give you pleasure or satisfaction, and then think about what else might be possible. Be creative in exploring ideas of other things you might enjoy. To begin with, the list may be very short, but you are likely to find that one idea leads on to another.

Anger

This is an emotion that is often felt by people with long-term illness. We talked about this in Chapter 9 on managing pain, but it is worth expanding on it. Loss, envy and frustration go with anger that what has happened is not fair. Anger often follows on from thoughts of injustice, of not being believed and of lack of recognition and understanding. These are some of the issues that we hear about most frequently:

- *Anger at the medical profession for not doing enough*—in recent times, we have come to believe that doctors can and should *cure* whatever is wrong with us, so it can come as an unpleasant shock to find that this is not always so. Very many of the long-term illnesses cannot be cured, though most can be treated and cared for.

- *Anger at lack of medical support*—you may feel angry because you believe that not enough is being done to help you. Provision of medical services for those with long-term illnesses is often patchy and limited.

- *Anger at lack of help from the community*—you may realize that you would cope better if you got more practical help. Even if some help is available, those who administer such services may do so in a way that makes a recipient feel demeaned at having to ask for help.

- *Anger at the 'unfairness' of it all*—people with long-term illness often feel anger because they can think of no reason why they deserve this fate.

- *Anger at some people's attitude to your illness*—we often hear of people's distress and anger as a response to things said to them about their illness by others, particularly when such remarks seem to be suggesting that they are, in some way, to blame for their illness.

- *Anger at those around you for not doing enough*—some people have wonderful family and friends who do a lot for them, but not everyone is so lucky. In any case, it is easy enough to feel that people could do more.

- *Anger about some trauma or accident that caused your long-term pain or disability.*

- *Old anger*—some of the problems you had before you were ill can still be with you. Some of the anger dating back years may be more noticeable today because now you are doing less you probably have less distraction from it.

Many people feel that they should not be angry, that it is wrong to have such feelings, but simply denying your anger does not usually help. You may have quite justifiable reasons for being angry. Anger can be a very positive emotion and move you to do something to right a wrong, or to stand up for your rights. However, it can also be a very damaging and fatiguing emotion and can alienate those who otherwise might help you. Acknowledging your own anger and the reasons for it can be an essential first stage in moving on. You can then explore the thinking behind your anger. If there is something you can fix, then fix it; if it cannot be fixed, then let it go.

Most of us seem to have an inbuilt sense of justice. We believe that life ought to be 'fair'. In fact, if we look around us we can see abundant evidence that life is frequently unfair. We can all see examples of 'bad' things happening to 'good' people. Concentrating on the 'unfairness' of what has happened to you is likely to increase your anger but unlikely to help you. Often, people know that they were 'injured' in some way and want those who caused the injury to acknowledge it and to apologize. They feel they are owed a debt. It is worth thinking about your particular 'injury'. Is it realistic to expect that, at this stage, you are going to get such an apology? If not, you might consider writing it off as a 'bad debt'. Who is suffering from your anger?

When I was a Credit Controller, there would sometimes be invoices that I could see were never going to be paid in spite of my best efforts. Rather than wasting my time and energy chasing them, I would get permission to write them off as a bad debt so that I could concentrate my efforts on invoices that I could get paid. Frankie

One of the things that can help fuel anger is poor communication. This is such an important subject that we deal with it much more fully in Chapter 24. If you can find ways of explaining the facts about your illness clearly and calmly, you may well reduce the aggravation you feel about other people's remarks and attitudes. If someone persists in a hurtful attitude in spite of being given the facts, that is really their problem—they obviously do not want to believe you. You may need to address that or even to end the relationship. It may help if you can bring yourself to feel pity for them for being so ignorant or prejudiced.

It is only too easy to feel that those around you could do more to help you, but you could explore the thinking behind this a bit more. Looking at it from their point of view may show you that they believe that they are already doing a lot and that what you are asking may, in their eyes, be too much. Perhaps you could try asking for help in a different way that does not suggest that you are taking them for granted.

If your illness was caused by some kind of trauma or injury, it is only human to look for someone who was responsible, someone to blame. Finding someone to blame, a scapegoat, may make you feel more comfortable, but it can also get in the way of thinking about what you can do to help yourself. Maybe our earlier notion of a 'bad debt', that is best written off, could apply here too.

Ask yourself 'Is my anger giving me any advantage? Is it helping me in any way?' If the answer is no, then acknowledge it and think what is behind it. Look at ways in which you could resolve the issue, choose not to dwell on it so much, or decide that such-and-such is really not worth going on being angry about. You may find that it helps if you find rituals that help you dispose of your anger—visualizing it being dropped into deep sea, writing about it and then screwing up the paper and throwing it in the waste paper basket, writing a letter to the person who offended you and then burning it. It is *your* anger, so you can choose what to do about it.

Feeling worried and anxious

Becoming ill is bound to produce problems and worries—such as how you are going to cope practically and financially, how long your illness will continue and whether you are going to get worse—to add to any worries you already had. Managing worry, not letting it get out of hand, is an important part of your self-help strategy.

Limiting your worry

In Chapter 11 on sleep problems, we talked about giving yourself a defined 'worry time'. What you need to avoid is thinking round and round your problems without resolving them. This is distressing, tiring and inefficient, and can spoil much of your time as well as making it more difficult to sleep well. If you can restrict your worry to a specific time each day, you are likely to be able to deal with it much more effectively. If a worry comes into your mind at another time, acknowledge it, and tell yourself that you will think about it during your worry time. Some people find that it helps if they make a note of it so that they can be confident that they will remember it and consider it later.

Keeping things in proportion

If you have many problems and worries, they can sometimes seem overwhelming. It is a common experience that when you are ill you view problems in a different way from the way that you did when you were well. A problem can seem bigger and more threatening. Talking things over with someone else can often enable you to get worries back into proportion. With each difficulty, could you stand back a little and say to yourself 'This is not a threat; it's just a problem. I'll deal with it now or later, but it won't help me to think about it all the time.'

Dealing with worry

You may decide to try the experiment of giving yourself a 'worry time'. If so, how can you use this time most effectively? It will certainly help if you are very structured in your approach to worry. Separate out your worries, being specific about what they are. Make a list, then deal with them *one at a time.* The techniques of 'problem solving' that we talk about in Chapter 16 will be useful in deciding what you can do about each worry. Accept that some problems cannot be solved immediately; if that is so, put those worries aside for the time being and concentrate on things that you can deal with now. Quite often, you will find that a worry looked at calmly during the day seems much less important than when it filled your mind during the night. So set a worry time, 'problem solve' one worry at a time, and enjoy the rest of your day.

Distraction

Finding ways of distracting yourself from worry can be helpful. This usually means doing something else or thinking about something else, so that you can stop thinking about the worry for a while and give yourself a break. Experiment with different types of distraction (doing something you enjoy or thinking about something else absorbing that will blot out the worry) and find out what works best for you.

Fear

Unfortunately, having a long-term illness can give rise to fear. You may be concerned that your condition could deteriorate, or may even know that that is very likely. You may realize that growing older will add to your difficulties. Your illness may have been successfully treated, but you can still have nagging fears about whether it will recur. A new symptom could be frightening. An increase in pain, fatigue or debility could leave you fearful of what that means. If your income has dropped because of your illness, you may have very justified concerns about how you are going to cope financially. There is a long list of things that you could fear without being unrealistic. Fear is a tiring emotion. It certainly can have a bad effect on your quality of life. So how do you deal with it?

Accept that you are afraid, without criticizing yourself for it. It is not a sign of moral weakness. It does not mean that you are a coward; it often means that you are realistic and brave. In our opinion, real courage is doing something in spite of being terrified. What you do with your fear and how you cope with it is the important thing.

Most fears are about something that might or will happen in the future. If you are accurate and realistic about what you fear, you may be able to make contingency plans about how you would deal with whatever might happen. The knowledge that you have a strategy to deal with a possible tomorrow can make things easier. Coming back into the present and dealing with what is happening today can help. Dealing with your present difficulties to the best of your abilities will give you confidence that you would deal well with extra problems that might occur in the future.

Fear can sometimes restrict you unnecessarily. You may be hesitant about doing certain things because you fear that they might do you harm or make your condition worse, which can restrict you and reduce your quality of life. Getting expert advice about what is possible (and perhaps desirable) in your condition can give you more confidence about trying things.

Of course, you are going to have times when you are very fearful about the future. Doing your best to limit the amount of time you spend thinking about your fears could be a very good thing. We suggested earlier that you give yourself a defined worry time. Could you do the same with fear? Do not spoil the present with fears of the future?

You may have a whole collection of fears, and worry about all of them, without considering that it is improbable that all of them will actually happen. Trying to cover all eventualities and giving yourself too much to think about does not help. It may be better to prioritize or to wait to see what actually does happen and deal with it then.

One of the biggest fears is that about death and dying. This is such an important subject that we look at it in more detail in Chapter 30.

Stress

Many people with a long-term illness find that stress makes them feel worse and so try to avoid it. However, it is not possible to avoid stress altogether, and trying to cut it out completely just does not work. You can work on both reducing the stress in your life and managing the inevitable remainder to make it less distressing. The techniques of 'problem solving' in Chapter 16 will be helpful. Relaxation and calm breathing can help to reduce the physical effects of stress on your body. Some of the stress in your life may be the result of poor communication between you and other people or between you and your doctor. In Chapters 24 and 27, we look at how you could address this problem.

You may need to look at what causes you stress and to think a bit about why this is. Talking it over with someone you trust can often help you to identify what stresses you most and then to find better ways of thinking about it or dealing with it.

Old problems

Some of the problems you had before you were ill may still be with you. You may even find that you have more time to notice them now you are ill.

Old anger, old grief, difficult relationships, and so on can add to present distress. Sometimes just bringing them out into the open and talking about them to a friend or relative can help, but you may decide that you would benefit from some professional help. This could be something to discuss with your doctor, who is likely to be able to point you in the right direction.

Low mood

Having a long-term illness can be distressing. It is not surprising if, at times, you find yourself in low spirits. Sometimes you are well aware of what has triggered off this state. It could be that something has happened that reminds you again of what you can no longer do. Perhaps someone, a doctor, a relation or a friend, has said something that has upset you. Maybe you are feeling lonely and isolated. Quite often though, the low mood can arrive with no obvious trigger. If fatigue is part of your package of symptoms, getting overtired can often leave you feeling miserable.

> If I find myself lying in bed leaking tears, it's usually because I've done too much. I can recognize this now and can comfort myself that it's just a symptom of my illness, and that this low mood will pass when I've had a good rest. Frankie

It can help if you can remind yourself that this mood is only temporary, particularly if you can do something to distract yourself, or if you accept that it is happening and give yourself a treat to reward yourself for coping with it.

Misery is usually transient. It can sometimes become persistent and become an illness—a depressive illness. There is more about this and how it can be helped in Chapter 22.

Loneliness and social isolation

This can be a major issue for some people. If you are restricted by your condition, whether because of fatigue or difficulties with mobility, having contact with other people can be difficult, and isolation and loneliness can be a real problem. Social contact is a very real human need; there are few of us who would be happy living like a hermit.

If your circumstances have changed because of your illness, you may find that some people who were good friends in the past seem to avoid you now. This is often because of their own difficulties, fears and embarrassment about illness; they do not necessarily believe that your illness is contagious, but in a superstitious way they somehow believe that your bad luck in becoming ill could be catching. Accept that that is their problem and not a reflection on you.

You may find that the ways in which you used to socialize are no longer possible. Going out with a crowd of friends for a drink may be too tiring. You may no longer meet people because of a common interest in activities such as sport. You may have lost the companionship of the workplace. Maybe the time has come to find a different kind of friend, or to socialize in a different kind of way. There are many kinds of ways of having social contact. Meeting just one person for a short time may suit you better now. You will probably find that you will have to take the initiative, rather than waiting for others to contact you. We talked more about this problem in Chapter 17.

Another way to deal with emotions

As well as doing something to lessen the emotions we have talked about, you could take another route. In your pre-illness life, you may have dealt with feeling bad by being very active, perhaps by doing something physical or by getting caught up in something that stopped you thinking about your emotions. That might have been effective, but it probably meant that you never did much to understand why you felt the way you did. If you are now stuck with your emotions and unable to escape from them in the old way, you could view this time as a positive opportunity to try something different.

You could experiment with just letting your feelings come into your mind and observing them dispassionately without getting sucked into thinking too much about them. For instance, when an emotion like anger comes into your mind, you could say to yourself 'Ah yes, I'm feeling angry. I'll just wait until it passes'. You do not need to condemn yourself for feeling that way or try to make the feeling disappear. You may well be surprised to find that emotions dealt with like that do pass. You can view them as visitors who do not have to be allowed to control you. This approach is part of the techniques of mindfulness meditation.

Cultivate your sense of humour

Humour really is important—and useful in managing your illness. Being able to see the funny side of things can help. If you can laugh at some of the things that happen in your illness, it can reduce the 'it's all so terrible' feelings. Laughter is a good medicine. Being able to laugh together is also a wonderful 'cement' in a relationship or in families. There is evidence that if you are smiling and not frowning, it is more difficult to think gloomy thoughts.

If you can show that you have a sense of humour, and that you can laugh at yourself as well as at funny things you are told, you are going to be a much nicer person to know than if you are gloomy most of the time. This can help you keep friends or make new ones. That will do a little to reduce any sense of social isolation.

Counselling

People who are finding coping emotionally with illness difficult often believe that counselling would be of value to them, but have a rather vague idea of how or why (or even what counselling is). As counselling may be expensive and/or for a limited number of sessions, it is sensible to think carefully about what you want from it before you start. A definite goal of 'I would like to be able to deal better with such-and-such' will enable you to get the most value from the counselling sessions. If you can select one or two topics that distress you the most, you can work on these with the counsellor. If you get those resolved, you can always move on to something else. Do your best to stick to your goal and not produce different issues at each session. There is more in Chapter 23 about how to choose a counsellor or therapist.

Further information

Manage Your Mind, Gillian Butler and Tony Hope.

22   Managing severe anxiety, panic or depression

We talked earlier about worry, fear and low spirits. States of overwhelming anxiety, panic and depression are severe versions of those emotions. You may have had a tendency to one or all of these states before you became ill, or it may be a very unwelcome extra now. They are all very unpleasant to experience and produce physical symptoms that add to the burden that illness has already placed on your body, so anything you can do (or can be helped to do) to control them will be of benefit to your general well-being.

Anxiety

Real anxiety can be more than just feeling a bit worried. For some people, it can mean waking up in the morning in a state of total dread, perhaps not even sure just what it is that is making them so anxious. Part of it is likely to be uncertainty about the future; part of it may be a feeling that their life is out of their control. Anything that can be done to identify the fears is likely to help. Bringing fears out into the open and then deciding what could be done to if the worst happened can give you more sense of control. You may find that when you have identified your fears, you can see that some of them are inaccurate, excessive or exaggerated.

Physical symptoms

One of the problems is that a state of anxiety can produce physical symptoms that make you feel even more unwell. This is another example of the effect of the mind on the body. These physical symptoms can add extra worries about whether your illness is getting worse, which can increase your anxiety. Physical symptoms of anxiety can include: palpitations; breathlessness; sweating; dry mouth; nausea; diarrhoea; twitching and shaking; muscle tension; and fatigue. Fast shallow breathing (hyperventilation) may be one of the things that add to the physical symptoms.

What helps?

See if you can establish that an increase in symptoms is due to anxiety and that when you are less anxious they subside. All the techniques of relaxation, calm breathing and distraction that we talked about earlier will help. Talking things over with someone you trust is also a good idea. Good research has shown that self-help techniques can be very effective.

Sometimes the level of anxiety is just too great for self-help to be enough. Getting professional help may be necessary. Your doctor or therapist may suggest that you try taking medicine for anxiety. Perhaps confusingly, the drugs called antidepressants are effective in reducing anxiety. You will certainly be helping your body if you give this a try. There is more about antidepressants later in the book. Tranquillizers can be useful for very short-term anxiety but are usually better avoided long term. You may also benefit from a form of cognitive behaviour therapy that has been specially developed to deal with anxiety. This is described in Chapter 23. One way or another, anxiety can be treated, so do not despair.

Panic

It can be terrifying to experience a panic attack—'an intense feeling of apprehension or impending doom, which is associated with a wide range of distressing physical symptoms'. These attacks may be so severe that those experiencing them fear that they are having a heart attack, that they will pass out or even die. As many panic attacks are associated with the fear of something dreadful happening when away from home, some people can also develop agoraphobia (a fear of leaving the safety of the home) which can be distressingly restrictive.

What helps?

One technique that may seem to help in the short term but actually makes things worse in the longer term is to avoid the problem—avoiding the places or the circumstances in which panic attacks are likely to happen. This may avoid panic attacks in the short term, but worsens the problem in the long term. Do your best not to avoid what you fear; instead work on managing the feelings of panic. There are techniques that have been proved to work.

- It is always easier to deal with panic as it is starting, rather that when it has built up into a full-blown panic attack. If you can recognize the early warning signs, you can start the techniques of relaxation and calm breathing that will damp down the physical reactions.

- Distraction—concentrating on something other than what you fear—can help.
- You can also become aware of what goes on in your mind during an attack. Look at some of these fears and check if they are really accurate. For example, is this chest pain really a heart attack? You have experienced this before and it went away after a while, leaving your heart perfectly healthy.

If you have frequent panic attacks, do get help from your doctor or from someone trained to deal with such things. Both psychological help and the drugs that are also used to treat depression can cure panic. You may be offered drugs such as beta blockers which can do something to damp down the physical symptoms that go with panic attacks. Help is available, so do ask for it.

Depression

Low mood some of the time is a normal reaction to illness. Learning how to manage your illness more actively may reduce your feelings of helplessness and hopelessness. Getting better at dealing with your problems will also give you a greater sense of control of your life.

However, if you find yourself feeling really low for much of the time, it is very important that you should get help. If you find yourself thinking seriously about suicide, you really do need to seek help. At this stage, it is not that important whether your depression is a reaction to the difficulties caused by your illness or whether you suffered from depression before you got ill. Just recognize it as something that can be treated.

What is depression?

Most people associate low mood with a 'depressive illness', but there are many other symptoms as well. In fact, it is possible to suffer from depression without feeling depressed! One key symptom is loss of interest, motivation and enjoyment (feelings called anhedonia). Depression can also show up as anxiety or extreme irritability. It can produce symptoms such as fatigue, pain, lack of energy or motivation, difficulty concentrating, reduced libido (sexual interest and drive), and lack of interest in food leading to weight loss.

If you suffer from depression, it does not mean that you are weak or pathetic—many notably gifted and heroic individuals suffer from episodes of depression. Winston Churchill used to call it his 'black dog'. Depression is not just all in the mind; there is evidence that it can also have a physical basis (an imbalance of neurotransmitters in the brain). Unfortunately, there is still a social stigma about any illness that can be thought of as 'mental', though this is getting much less. Do your best not to be ashamed of it. It can be tempting to think 'I'm not the sort of person to get depressed', but do you really know who does get depressed? Accept that it is an extra burden for you now, but one that you can do something about and that can be treated. Be tolerant of family and friends if they find it easier to deny your depression.

Seasonal affective disorder

Some people find that their mood gets worse in the autumn and improves in the spring. It may be that they are suffering from what is called seasonal affective disorder (SAD). It is possible that seeing less sunlight during the winter months has an effect on parts of the brain. Some sufferers have found that regular use of a light box (sitting in front of a very bright light for several hours a day) can be helpful. However, it is a time-consuming and cumbersome remedy—taking a suitable antidepressant drug may be a more practical option.

Antidepressant drugs

Your doctor may suggest that you try an antidepressant. You may well have some concerns about taking such drugs. It could be helpful if we look more closely at some of these concerns.

- Some people simply dislike the idea of taking these drugs, feeling that they should be able to manage their problems themselves. This is an entirely understandable and laudable view but, although antidepressants will not change your problems, they can help you to a state in which you are better able to deal with them. You do not have to think in terms of drugs *or* self-help. You can use both.

- Others feel that their condition is not really depression and that therefore an antidepressant is not an appropriate drug. However, these drugs can help a variety of conditions, not just depression. They can help with pain, fatigue, sleep disturbance and other symptoms. Rather than worry about the name, it may be better to give it a go and see if it helps.

- Many people think that antidepressant drugs may be addictive or cause long-term harm. This is understandable, given the reputation of the tranquillizing benzodiazepines such as diazepam (Valium) for being addictive and producing very nasty withdrawal symptoms when stopped. Although some of the newer antidepressant drugs may cause some increase in symptoms if they are stopped suddenly, this is uncommon if they are withdrawn slowly and carefully.

How to take an antidepressant

All effective drugs have some side effects, and antidepressants are no exception. Some people get noticeable side effects, but others do not. Starting with a small dose and building up gradually will minimize the chance that you will get bad side effects. However, it is important to remember that to treat depression you will probably have to work up to a full effective dose (sometimes called the therapeutic dose) as recommended by your doctor. The danger of only trying these drugs at a low dose is that you could end up rejecting something as ineffective which might have been very helpful at a higher dose.

One of the curious things about antidepressants is that they take a while to become effective. Although you may benefit almost immediately from a sedative effect, you are quite likely to notice side effects *before* you feel other benefits. Most of these drugs do not start to have beneficial effects on energy and mood for at least 2–4 weeks after starting to take them at a therapeutic dose. Be prepared for a period during which you experience side effects but not much benefit. Do your best to stick it out. It is bad enough being ill without feeling miserable as well!

There is a general agreement that a fair trial of these drugs is 6 weeks at full dose. Clearly, if the benefits do not outweigh the disadvantages at this stage, it is a good idea to talk to your doctor about stopping the drug. If possible, it would be better to reduce the dose gradually, rather than stopping abruptly.

Choosing an antidepressant

Antidepressants require a prescription. Your doctor will therefore guide you in which drug to take. An experienced doctor or psychiatrist can select the drug that is most suitable for you. Some are good at reducing pain. Some have a sedating effect, which can be helpful if you are having problems with sleep. Others are somewhat energizing, which can be helpful if you have problems getting going in the morning or in motivating yourself to action. Some drugs seem to have more effect on anxiety. There is no single drug that works the best for everyone. It is very much a matter of 'horses for courses'.

The different types of antidepressants

There are four main types of antidepressants that are commonly used to treat depression, though other drugs are used as well

- The tricyclics—the advantage of these is that they have been used by millions of patients for half a century, so a lot is known about them. They are effective and we can be reasonably sure that they have no long-term harmful effects. The main disadvantage is that they are harmful in overdose and they do tend to cause some degree of side effects—the principal ones being a dry mouth, reduction in the ability of the eye to cope with bright lights at night, and sometimes a tremor. They can also increase appetite, which is good if you have lost too much weight, but not so good if you do not want to put weight on. Other possible side effects will be listed in the packet the drug comes in. Do remember that the manufacturers are required to list all possible side effects—you will probably not get most of them. Most of these drugs are sedative, so taken at night they can aid sleep.

- The SSRIs—selective serotonin reuptake inhibitors (SSRIs) are the most commonly prescribed antidepressants. They are as effective as the older drugs, but are much safer in overdose and have fewer side effects. However, they may not be as effective in reducing pain. The principal side effect is nausea.

- The newer agents—pharmaceutical companies are continually striving to develop more effective drugs that work rapidly and have few side effects. The advantage of these is that they represent the pinnacle of pharmaceutical development, but one potential disadvantage is that we cannot yet be as certain that there are no long-term effects. An important category is the dual action agents such as Venlafaxine. These combine properties of tricyclics and SSRIs. They are useful. They are as effective as the older drugs, but are much safer in overdose. They have fewer side effects and reduce pain.

- There are also a number of less frequently used drugs such as the MAOIs (monoamine oxidase inhibitors). If you are prescribed one of these, discuss the advantages and disadvantages with your doctor.

Multiple drugs

Doctors will sometimes give drugs in combination to people who do not respond to taking a single one. Combining drugs may increase the risk of serious side effects so is usually only done on the advice of specialists. One potentially useful combination is a non-sedative drug in the morning and a sedative one at night. Such combinations should only be used under the supervision of a doctor.

Herbal antidepressants

People who dislike taking the products of the pharmaceutical industry for whatever reason sometimes prefer herbal preparations that are claimed to be antidepressant. One such preparation is 'St John's Wort' (*Hypericum perforatum*). There is some evidence that this herb has an action similar to the antidepressants described above. Even though it is considered more natural, some people do experience side effects from it. It can also conflict with some prescribed drugs, so you should always check with your doctor or pharmacist before taking it. This apparently 'natural' alternative does also have a significant disadvantage. It can be hard to judge the quality and the quantity of what you are taking. Whatever one thinks about the pharmaceutical companies, they produce drugs of great purity in very carefully controlled doses. It is very much harder to do this with herbal preparations.

Non-drug treatments

Some people prefer not to take drugs or find that they are unable to tolerate the side effects of antidepressants, even if they start them off very slowly. This does *not* mean that there is nothing that can be done to treat their depression. There are other ways of tackling the problem. Cognitive behaviour therapy (CBT) was first developed as a treatment for depression, though it is now used for many other illnesses too. CBT for depression aims to help you become aware of and to change the inaccurate and overly negative thoughts that are 'pushing mood down'. It is a collaborative process between a patient and a therapist. Many research trials have shown that for mild to moderately severe depression, it can be as effective a treatment as antidepressant drugs. We talk about this more in Chapter 23. Although it is very much easier to use CBT with a trained therapist, it is possible to do a good deal of this by yourself.

Other things can help too. One of the things that can trigger depression is to find yourself in a very difficult, distressing situation over which you have no control (which could be a description of your own illness state). That is just one of the reasons that self-management can be so important—it can give you back a sense of control. Research has shown that practising 'problem solving' (see Chapter 16) can help with depression. Finding someone who will listen to you is always helpful, particularly if they understand about depression. You really can believe that this black patch will pass and that you will come out on the other side.

Rumination

If you suffer anxiety, panic or depression, there is a risk of falling victim to rumination—going over and over problems in your mind. This will only make you feel worse. Recognize when you are doing this and do something to help you break away from it. If it is possible, find something enjoyable, but anything else that works will do—even if it is something as meaningless as counting the spots on the wallpaper!

Further information

Manage Your Mind, Gillian Butler and Tony Hope.

Overcoming Anxiety, Helen Kennerly.

Panic Attacks, Christine Inghams.

Overcoming Depression, Paul Gilbert.

23 Getting psychological help

You are not alone if you have some emotional problems as well as physical ones; a large proportion of people with a long-term illness suffer in this way. Such problems might have been there before you became ill, or they could be a reaction to the difficulties, distress and losses associated with your illness. Getting help with your emotional problems could do a lot to improve your quality of life now. Such things as anxiety or depression can be very distressing and can add physical symptoms to those caused by your illness.

You may feel reluctant to admit to emotional problems, particularly if your illness is one that does not have a clear medical label or diagnosis. You may fear that your doctor will think that this is proof that your illness is 'all in the mind'. Though this fear is understandable, it is actually a poor reason for denying yourself the help you need. Could you try to overcome your reluctance and seek help?

So what help could you look for? Just having someone you trust, whether a member of your family or a good friend, and talking things over with them can be really helpful. Putting your problems or distress into words can make it easier for you to see what you could do about it. Sometimes, though, this is not enough, in which case looking for professional assistance could be a good idea. There are three areas in which you might find such assistance—the health service, the voluntary sector or a therapist whom you pay privately.

Therapy obtained through the health service may well be time limited and you may have to join a long waiting list to get it. Your family doctor is usually the gatekeeper to such services. There may be a counsellor attached to your practice, or you may need to be referred elsewhere. Depending on your particular illness, there may be counselling offered through your hospital clinic. Unfortunately, some people are reluctant to involve their doctor, perhaps fearing the consequences of having a referral to mental health services on their medical record.

You may be able to get some help from the voluntary sector, for example from organizations such as Relate, The Samaritans or Cruse. You may find that there is a local service offering psychological help that does not require a referral from a doctor.

There are a great many private therapists. Whether you choose to use one of them can depend on your financial situation, though you may have medical insurance which covers treatment by a psychiatrist or psychologist. Costs can vary. Some therapists may offer a reduced rate to people on benefit, but this is not the norm. If you do choose to go down this route, you would have more choice, and could pick someone you find compatible. Finding someone who suits your style can make the process of therapy somewhat easier. A personal recommendation can be helpful. Your doctor may know of someone suitable. If you cannot get such a recommendation, you can find lists of local therapists in the telephone Yellow Pages directory. See if you can talk to a therapist either in person or on the phone before you agree to work with them. You have a right to ask about their qualifications, what the cost of sessions would be and how long they would be likely to continue. Such a conversation could give you a feeling about the therapist and whether he or she seems compatible.

Different therapies

There are different kinds of psychological help you may be offered or seek out for yourself. Knowing a bit about the different types could help you in making a choice.

We start off by looking at cognitive behavioural therapy (CBT) as this form of help has been most widely used and researched in helping people with long-term illnesses. Many of the self-help books we recommend are based on CBT principles and techniques. Unfortunately, there are not enough trained CBT therapists available in many areas. Do not despair though; self-help using such books can also be effective.

Cognitive behavioural therapy (CBT)

The term cognitive behavioural therapy sounds very technical and very psychological. It is not really either. It is actually advanced common sense. It is based on the ways in which physicians have tried to help their patients for more than a hundred years. The modern therapy that is called CBT was developed over 30 years ago by an American psychiatrist Aaron Beck as a treatment for depression. Since then, it has been adapted to treat many other conditions, both psychological and physical. There is a substantial body of research evidence that demonstrates its effectiveness, and its principles form the mainstay of most chronic illness management programmes.

CBT for depression

People suffering from depression are typically low in mood. They also tend to have negative and inaccurate thoughts and beliefs, thinking negatively about themselves (I'm useless), their circumstances (it's awful) and their future (it's hopeless). This distorted thinking was long thought to be simply a *result* of their depression. Beck's innovation was to suggest and demonstrate that this thinking could also be a *cause* of their depression and that, by changing their thinking, patients could get better.

CBT works by helping patients to develop more accurate and helpful ways of thinking about themselves, their situation and their future. This does not mean adopting equally inaccurate positive thinking, but rather getting evidence by testing out alternative thoughts and beliefs to see which reflect the real world in the most accurate way.

During the treatment sessions, the therapist helps the patients to clarify how they are thinking and coping now and to consider different ways of thinking and behaving. Between treatment sessions, patients carry out 'homework' tasks. For instance, they may be set the task of catching and recording their thoughts about themselves such as 'I am a failure'. Once these thoughts have been identified, the patient can be helped to challenge them by looking at alternative views (e.g. 'some of the things I have tried to do have failed, but others have succeeded. This does not make me a failure as a person.') Finally, the evidence for each is examined (by reviewing past achievements, asking other people or trying out new endeavours).

CBT for anxiety, panic and phobias

Once the value of CBT in depression was established, psychiatrists and psychologists went on to identify inaccurate and distorted thinking in patients with other problems such as anxiety, panic and phobias. For example, people suffering from anxiety tend to exaggerate their fears; people who panic tend to 'catastrophize' physical symptoms (a twinge of chest pain is interpreted as 'I am having a heart attack') and consequently pay excessive attention to minor bodily symptoms. A person with phobia tends to exaggerate risk (e.g. someone who fears flying may think 'there is a 90% chance that this plane will crash' and consequently avoid flying).

Versions of CBT were developed to help patients overcome such problems. Again, these are based on identifying the thoughts and the ways of thinking associated with such problems, and then finding more realistic alternatives. Patients are encouraged to challenge negative thoughts and catastrophic interpretations of symptoms.

CBT for physical illnesses

In recent years, forms of CBT have been developed for people suffering from a wide range of physical conditions such as chronic pain and the after effects of a heart attack. Using CBT, patients can be helped to cope most effectively, to improve their ability to function and their quality of life.

After an initial assessment, the therapist and patient together might look at such things as:

- re-evaluation of illness beliefs (rather than saying 'this belief is inaccurate', the therapist would encourage the patient to try some behavioural experiments to check the accuracy of such beliefs for themselves and then look at other possible beliefs.)
- stabilizing activity/rest/sleep
- an experiment of a gradual increase in activity
- reviewing unhelpful attitudes
- problem solving practical difficulties
- reviewing and planning for the future.

Summary

CBT seeks to help individuals to find the best ways of managing their illness to produce an increased quality of life and have a good chance of decreasing disability. It also helps patients to identify and deal with 'what gets in the way of being sensible'. It is a 'tool', not a rigid form of treatment. It can be adapted to an individual's needs and concentrate on the areas that will produce the most benefit for that individual—whether a physical improvement or an increase in their quality of life.

Does CBT help people with long-term conditions?

Yes, it does seem to help. It is not a cure, but research trials, clinical experience and anecdotal evidence have shown that it can help patients with long-term illness to cope better, to manage medical treatment better, to have fewer symptoms and to have a better quality of life.

Other psychotherapies

Different styles of therapy may be more suitable for some people:

Psychodynamic therapy is based on the ideas of Freud, who developed an approach based on listening to patients' history in depth. He believed that only by discovering the origins of their problems in earlier experience would cure be possible. Modern therapy is based more on working on current relationships and how they may be adversely affected by previous experiences.

Cognitive analytical therapy uses a cognitive approach to analyse earlier events and their influence on current feelings and behaviours.

Interpersonal therapy (IPT) uses cognitive, behavioural and psycho-dynamic concepts and techniques to focus on the patient's relationships and the problems arising from them.

In addition to the 'formal' psychotherapies described above, *simple psychotherapies* are important too. They merge imperceptibly into the therapeutic component of all doctor–patient relationships.

Counselling is a loosely defined activity whereby people are helped to cope with, or overcome, problems in their lives. The counsellor serves as a support, a facilitator of emotional expression, a source of information, and as someone off whom ideas can be bounced. Counselling is provided in many settings, mostly non-psychiatric.

Problem solving therapy is a simple but effective practical treatment to help the people identify and solve problems in their lives. It is often used as part of CBT. We talked about this technique in Chapter 16.

Supportive psychotherapy describes the supportive element of a therapist–patient relationship. All health care workers—as well as relatives and friends—provide supportive psychotherapy to some degree whether they realize it or not. It does not aim to produce change, but to help people to cope with adversity or other problems, often over a sustained period.

Group therapy originated from the view that it is helpful for patients to share experiences and feelings. It may be based on CBT or on other types of therapy. It suits some people well, but not others.

In summary, there are many labels and variations of therapy. All are merely descriptions of ways in which one person can help another cope better with life and illness. They are all based on the idea that we can all benefit from reflecting on how we deal with problems in our life, under-standing ourselves better and trying out new ways of doing things.

Further information

The Which? Guide to Counselling and Therapy.

section 4
Managing interpersonal problems

24 Relationships and communication

The relationships that we have with the people around us are a vital part of our lives; this is especially true if you have a long-term illness. Good relationships can make all the difference to the way people cope with their illness and to their quality of life. Unfortunately, being ill can change these relationships. Even the best relationship can be put under strain and one that was a little rocky to begin with may become even more difficult.

A difficult relationship, with a partner, family, friends, doctors or officials, is an obvious source of stress, and will not be helpful to you in managing your condition, so anything you can do to ease or improve the relationship will be of benefit to you.

In the following sections, we look at a variety of things that have been proved to help, though, as always, we stress that there are no absolute rules—each person and each relationship is different. However, we hope that some of the ideas may be helpful to you.

Better communication

Good communication is the basis of a good relationship, so this seems like the best place to start. One of the things that can add to the difficulty of managing any long-term illness is poor communication with the people around you. Getting a message across clearly and calmly can do a lot to make a difficult situation easier. Even if you think that this is not one of your natural abilities, good communication is only a skill and, like any skill, it can be learned. Here are some aspects of communication that we think are particularly relevant to a person with a long-term illness.

Quiet assertiveness

It is all too easy to slip into the trap of feeling that you have stopped having rights since you became ill. Perhaps you have had to stop working and no longer feel like a productive member of society, or perhaps you now have to accept help when once you did things for yourself. Your image of yourself may have changed for the worse. This sort of thing can make you feel diminished and less of a real person. People around you can sometimes behave towards you in ways that seem to reinforce this belief. It is important for you to believe that you *do* still have rights, no more and no less than the people around you, even if you cannot do all that you once did. You will communicate better if you can be quietly assertive, but that assertiveness has to be based on the belief that you still have rights.

It can be very helpful to think about what your rights are now, taking your illness into account. What rights would you give to someone else in your own circumstances? This is a list of rights that may give you some useful ideas for yourself:

I believe that I have the right:

- to ask anyone for anything, whilst respecting their right to say no
- to say no myself without feeling guilty
- to look after myself and not to be pushed into doing something that might jeopardize my health and well-being
- to enjoy myself
- to have different levels of abilities depending on the fluctuations in my illness
- to choose what help I will accept
- to be consulted about decisions that will affect me
- to choose whether or not to be involved in someone else's problems
- to give as well as to receive
- to have emotions and to mind about what has happened to me
- to change
- to be confused
- to be kind and forgiving to myself when I make mistakes
- not to feel guilty about being ill
- to believe that being is as important as doing.

Balance your rights against the rights of the people around you. It is a two-way process. Other people have rights that need to be thought about too.

Having read this list, could you make one of your own that takes account of your particular circumstances, and with which you feel comfortable? You might find writing it down helpful. You could then use it to reinforce yourself when you have moments of self-doubt.

If you can be quietly confident in yourself as a person with rights, then you will find it much easier to talk to other people and to be taken seriously.

Belated fluency

The French have a phrase 'esprit de l'escalier'—the humour of the staircase—which refers to the witty remark that a person thinks of only after leaving the party and going down the stairs. Thinking, after the event, of something that could have been said is something that happens to all of us, but it can be particularly irritating in encounters relating to illness. Thinking too late of the question you should have asked the doctor, or the reply you could have made to someone who said something stupid about your illness, can leave you feeling frustrated and cross. Instead of just cursing, it is a good idea to write down what you might have said. That way you are likely to remember it in similar circumstances. If you can build up an anthology of good ways of putting things, you are much more likely to be able to express yourself better another time. You could add to your list something that someone else has said that strikes you as a good way of putting things, or something you have read that expresses an aspect of your illness rather well.

Preparing for an encounter or an interview by thinking about what needs to be said or the questions that need to be asked will help. It is often sensible to write a list beforehand to help you to remember.

Explaining an invisible illness

A great many long-term illnesses are invisible; they often have few outward signs. Pain, malaise and fatigue do not necessarily show. People tend to judge you by what they see of you, particularly if they only meet you when you are feeling well enough to get out or to receive visitors. They often do not see the times when you are at your worst.

People can be remarkably ignorant about illness. (How much did you know about your own illness before you got it?) You cannot expect them to understand what it is like for you unless they are given the facts. It is worth checking up on what they do know and then filling in the gaps. You may choose not to tell some people about your illness, but you then have to accept that, if you do not tell them, they are likely to think of you as a well person.

If when somebody asks you how you are, you automatically answer 'fine', then fine is how people are going to think you are. That may be how you want most people to consider you, but it can lead to misunderstanding and irritation too. You may need to think of something you could answer that is a bit more accurate, without going into too much detail about your state of health. You do not need to stress how terrible things are. See if you can find a good balance between too little and too much.

If I am asked how I am, I often reply 'I'm surviving, but how are **you**?' which indicates I've got something to survive, but which doesn't burden the person I'm talking to. Frankie

Those with an illness often want *all* of those around them to understand *all* about their condition. This is unrealistic, but a more specific approach is not. Think about just one person and one thing you would like them to understand. Then try asking yourself these questions:

- What particular aspect of your illness do you want then to understand?
- What information would help them understand?
- What would they be saying or doing that would show that they did understand?
- Is what you want something they can give?
- Is it reasonable to expect them to give it to you?

Once you have got that clear in your mind, you can start thinking about what information to give them and how to explain your reasonable needs. It may take time for them to adjust to this approach.

Talking to yourself

You may find it strange to find this in a section on communication, but there is a point to it—you are the most important person you talk to. The way you communicate with yourself, the language you use about yourself (even in your thoughts), can make a lot of difference to how you feel about yourself. Being really honest with yourself and putting your thoughts into words, rather than just being aware of the emotions they produce, will help you understand why you feel as you do, and what may need to change for you to feel better. Someone once said 'I don't know what I think until I hear myself saying it'. Even if you do not admit all of your feelings about what is happening to you to those around you, it is important that you admit them to yourself.

Be kind and gentle with yourself. You might be telling yourself things that you would find insulting if they came from someone else. You might say things like 'I'm so stupid', 'I'm being a wimp' or 'I'm being pathetic'. Notice that these are generalizations. It is more helpful and accurate to think in specifics. For example, you may at times be a bit silly and not manage yourself as well as you could; that does not make you stupid. Having to let other people do some things for you does not make you a wimp. Feeling sorry for yourself at times does not make you pathetic.

Beware of absolutist thinking. People often use very absolutist language about themselves such as 'I'll *never* get this right.' 'I *always* make mistakes.', when the reality is that getting it right might take some time, or that they sometimes make mistakes. Do you recognize any of this in yourself? If so, this is a good time to start catching yourself up when you hear yourself saying this sort of thing, and rephrasing it in a way that is more accurate (and kinder to yourself).

What exactly you mean when you say 'I can't'? It would be accurate to say that you cannot jump a 10 foot fence, but often people mean things like 'I really don't want to do such-and such', 'I'm frightened that doing such-and such would make me worse', 'I haven't done such-and-such before and I'm not certain that I'd be successful'. Saying 'I can't do such-and-such' can lead you to believe that it is impossible and this can be very restrictive. Keep 'can't' for what is really impossible and explore the possibility that actually you can.

Asking for help

Many people find it difficult to ask for help. Sometimes they feel that they *ought* to be able to cope on their own and that it is a sign of weakness to have to ask. Sometimes they feel diminished by having to ask. Often they fear rejection. 'What if he or she said no!' It is worth thinking about your own feelings about this. If someone in your position asked you for something that was within your power to give without too much trouble, would you turn them down, or think less of them for asking? As long as what you ask for is reasonable, most people do not mind being asked, particularly if you can make it clear that you would not be offended by a refusal. A good working motto is 'I have a right to ask anyone for anything, as long as I respect their right to say no'. Inevitably, some people will turn you down, but that does not make you less of a person. It may well be that their refusal is to do with their own feelings about illness, or because of something that is going on in their lives that you do not know about. Maybe they are just plain selfish, in which case they are probably not the sort of friends you need now.

People may sometimes offer the kind of help that they believe you need, even when it is not something you want. You have a perfect right to refuse it. One way to do this is to thank them for their offer and then suggest something different that you do want.

Just saying no

If someone does not know the details of your illness, they may ask you to do things for them or with them that would be too much for you or inappropriate in your condition. Whilst you have the right not do what they ask, many people find refusing difficult. One approach that may help is to thank the person asking you before saying no. Alternatively, you can turn down the whole request with a genuine show of regret, but to offer to do something smaller instead.

Improve your listening skills

Good communication is a two-way process. You will not communicate well if you do not really hear what the other person is saying. So working on your listening skills will help. Some useful tips might be:

- Give the other person time to put their point across. Try not to interrupt or finish their sentences for them.
- Show that you have heard what they are saying by picking up a point they have made and repeating it or paraphrasing it.
- If you did not understand what they meant, ask them to explain it further.
- As well as listening carefully, watch their body language. That may show you more about how they are feeling.

Some other practical suggestions

Here are some suggestions for better communication:

- Try to stay calm. If you express strong emotion, other people may discount much of what you say 'She doesn't really mean that; she's just angry. She'll be more reasonable when she's calmed down'. This is particularly true when talking to young people; emotion in a parent seems to produce selective deafness in teenagers! Anger certainly gets in the way.
- Keep it short and simple. Long-winded explanations often make people lose interest.
- If possible, try to tap into the experience of the person you are talking to. For instance, if you are trying to explain the overwhelming exhaustion you may experience, try reminding them of a time when they experienced something similar (like reminding a mother of what it was like when she had a teething baby keeping her awake at night, as well as an active toddler to care for during the day). When you have explained the

similarities, you can outline the differences—for example, it may not take much to get you exhausted and a 'good night's sleep' may not make you feel much better. If you are trying to explain your malaise, you could remind them of the way they felt the last time they had a really bad bout of flu.

- Try to stand back and look at things from the other person's point of view. That may show you that they are not being quite as unreasonable as you first believed. If you feel you have good cause to complain about what they are doing (or not doing), try to stick to criticisms of their actions, not of them as people.

- Do your best to stay consistent, even though your illness may fluctuate. Try not to turn down help crossly one day when you are feeling a bit better and then be wounded another time because help is not offered. It is better to say something like 'Thank you so much for offering, but I feel well enough do it today. I do enjoy doing things for myself when I can. I'll certainly ask you to help another time if I don't think I can manage it.'

- Even if you hate having to feel grateful, saying 'thank you' always helps. It can help if you can explain how and why something done for you has been helpful, or to say how well the job has been done.

- Think about your body language. Does it express what you want to convey?

- Give them something simple to read to explain your illness. Hospital clinics and the self-help patient organizations often have suitable leaflets.

Planning is often useful. If you have something important to say, a specific point you want to make, it is often helpful to think about it and to write it down in advance. That way you can be certain that you will say exactly what you mean. This can be particularly important when talking to doctors or officials. There is more about this later in the section on your relationship with your doctor.

Further information

Manage Your Mind, Gillian Butler and Tony Hope—Chapters 13 and 15.
Living a Healthy Life with Chronic Conditions, Kate Lorig—Chapter 10.

25 Caring and being cared for

A long-term illness affects both the carer and the person being cared for. It can change both their lives. It may help to think of it as a new joint project that can bring positive as well as negative things to both of you.

It is not always easy either caring or being cared for. Both sides can be dealing with loss, resentment (even if it is not expressed) and difficulties. A carer may have had to give up important areas of his or her life to allow them to care; the person cared for may have had to give up independence as well as carrying their burden of illness. So it is a particular type of relationship that needs special attention. Whilst the amount of care needed and the time involved will vary with the severity of the illness and the disability it causes, the dynamic is that one person needs care and the other person is giving it.

Finding the right balance between the wants and needs of these two people is not easy. For instance, the carer may want to get things done smoothly and quickly, while the person cared for may want to retain as much independence as possible, which can slow things down. To give an example:

Anna is a woman with rheumatoid arthritis who walks very slowly. Her husband Bill would like her to use a wheelchair while they are out shopping so that they could get things done faster, which would leave more time for him to do the things he wants. Anna really dislikes the thought of being seen in a wheelchair and being thought of as a cripple.

One can have sympathy for both of them. There is no absolute right or wrong answer to the problem; often the best solution is some kind of a compromise.

Being a carer

If you are looking after someone who is ill, you are doing a very important job. It is unfortunate that in our society carers often do not get the recognition they deserve. They frequently do not get the back-up and help that would make their lives easier, although there may be some help available if you keep on asking for it. Of course, the degree of care you need to give can vary enormously, and your need for help varies accordingly. There is more about getting practical help in Chapter 29.

Do you feel guilty that you are not caring in a perfect way? You need not; nobody can be a perfect carer all of the time. It is much better that you are doing the job, however imperfectly, than that it is not being done at all. It is only human that at times you may feel frustration, resentment and anger. However much you love the person you are caring for, there are bound to be times when compassion fatigue sets in. The illness may have changed them, so that they are now a very different person from the one you first knew. It can be helpful to have somebody with whom you can discuss these issues, without feeling that you are being disloyal. Carer support groups are available in most areas; why not use them? They may be a valuable source of information and help. It can be a great release to be able to talk to other people who are experiencing the same kind of difficulties as you are. If you do not want to talk, writing down your feelings can be a release.

Much as I loved my husband, there were times when I longed to scream at him. He could be really pig headed in refusing to cooperate in things that would have made my life easier. At times I thought about saying things like 'For goodness sake, pull yourself together. Don't be such a wimp. I know you are going through a hard time, but it's not easy for me either.' Mostly I just thought those things, but I still felt guilty. Frankie

Other people may express sympathy for the person who is ill, but they often do not acknowledge your difficulties as a carer, so that you can be left feeling 'but what about me? I'm being brave too. I deserve some praise'.

It can be very tempting to try to take over completely and run things your way. That can certainly make things easier at times, but it is not good for the person you care for. You can make things too easy for them. They need to retain some degree of independence. They need to be allowed to do things in their own way, at least some of the time, and to make their own mistakes. There has to be a balance.

Looking after a child

Caring for a child with a long-term illness can be particularly painful and distressing. Although we do not cover childhood illnesses specifically in this book, much of what we say, including all that we have said about searching for information and support, also applies to children. As a carer, you will have to use your own judgement as to what you can get from this book and what else you will need to find.

Look after your own needs

It is not selfish to consider your own needs. Some time off from caring is vital. It may be difficult to arrange if you need to provide 24 hour cover, but it is worth striving for. Explore respite care, even if it is only for a short time. Could the person you care for go to a day centre one or two days a week? Could you find someone who would come in for a while so that you could get out on your own? You really do need to have some life of your own, aside from being a carer, and you will be a better carer for it.

If you have had to give up your job, you might do something towards keeping up your old skills, or maybe learning some new ones. For instance, if you are not computer literate, this could be a very good time to learn how to use one. A computer can give you access to helpful sources of information and be a good way to keep in touch with friends via e-mail, or to make new contacts. Getting in touch with a chat room dedicated to a particular illness could offer a whole new type of support.

It is important to look after yourself both physically and emotionally. Your health is vital to both of you. If you have to do lifting, get expert advice on to how to do it in the safest way. Back trouble is the last thing you need now. Your own self-esteem can be undermined by what you are going through. It is only too easy to feel that you have become a non-person since you became a carer. Remind yourself that you are doing something very valuable. There are bound to be times when you are under a lot of stress. Look at all the ways in which you could manage your stress, so that it does not overwhelm you.

Helpful equipment

There may well be equipment that would make your life easier. Some may be quite cheap and within your budget to purchase. Things such as grab rails might be installed for you. Other more expensive things might be available on loan. Research what would help and where you might get it. A home visit from an occupational therapist would mean that you get really expert advice. A local carers' support group will probably be able to help too.

Stresses within the family

A particularly difficult situation can be when one member of a family is expected to care for a parent or parents, and that person receives very little help from the other siblings. We hear about this very often. This can produce anger and resentment, with strong feelings of injustice. Whether anything can be done to improve the situation depends very much on the dynamics within the family, but it is usually of some help if the carer can negotiate *some* assistance from siblings and is open about his or her feelings.

The end of caring

Something that may need to be considered is what happens if the person you care for goes into long-term residential care, or sadly if they die. In these circumstances you may suddenly find yourself without your accustomed role and feel very lost. That is just one reason for maintaining some kind of independent life of your own. People tell us how difficult it can be to get back to ordinary living again. There may also be financial problems when the benefits that may have formed a significant part of your income are withdrawn. It does no harm, and may do some good, to do some forward planning.

> It certainly made things a little easier for me after my husband died that I had some independent life of my own through writing and doing telephone counselling. Frankie

Caring at a distance

So far we have talked about caring for someone living with you, but an increasingly common situation is the need to arrange care for someone (usually a parent) who is not geographically close. This can be extremely difficult and can mean that very hard choices have to be made. Should you move to be closer to them, or should you relocate the relative to be closer to you? If you have arranged care for them where they now live, how can you check that the care is adequate and suitable? This is a huge subject, but we can recommend some very helpful books.

Further information

The Selfish Pig's Guide to Caring, Hugh Marriott
Caring for Someone at a Distance, AGE Concern.

Being cared for

It is not easy being a carer, but it can be just as difficult having to be cared for. It can be both frustrating and irritating having to accept help with things that you used to be able to do for yourself. As we said earlier, it may help if you see this as a joint project in which you are both equally involved. If your condition fluctuates, there may be times when you can do some things and other times when those are impossible. This can be confusing for your carer, who may end up feeling that they are always doing the wrong thing. You might try talking about this and find ways of indicating when you need help and when you do not. Do your best not to seem to be blaming your carer. Maybe this is an area in which structured 'problem solving' (see Chapter 16) would be useful.

One of the sources of difficulty can be insisting on going on doing something for yourself, even if it leaves you feeling exhausted and miserable. It might be easier for your carer if you could accept help gracefully. You might be very much better tempered if you did not wear yourself out. This is an area in which you should keep reviewing the situation and learning how to accept different forms of help.

Managing your emotions

If you are suffering from a long-term illness, there are likely to be times when you are feeling angry or frustrated. It can be very tempting to take your emotions out on whoever is nearest, which will usually be your carer. This may leave you feeling a little better, but does nothing for the relationship. Could you find other ways of letting off steam? We talked earlier of the difficulties of being a carer, and these do need to be considered. Try imagining yourself in their place and seeing things from their point of view. Your own life will be better if you can work on keeping the relationship easy and smooth.

Think about your carer's needs too

Carers have a real need for some time to themselves. They are not being heartless or selfish to want this. It will be much better if you can accept this gracefully and even encourage them in it. You may not enjoy being left on your own, or having to accept some stranger looking after you for a while, but it will make things much easier in the long run. There might be a day centre that you could attend sometimes. You might not enjoy this much, but it could be a welcome break for your carer. You could see all this as one of your contributions to the success of the relationship.

Keep working on the relationship between you and your carer

Keep reminding yourself that you are still a worthwhile person, even though you are ill. You have a right to be consulted about what happens to you and what decisions are made about you. You have rights, but so does your carer. It is when there is a balance between the two that things are most likely to work out well.

Good communication is vital. It is a great mistake to think 'but they *ought* to understand'. Spell things out calmly and clearly to them. Say what aspects of your care you find difficult. Let your carer do the same. Together, you may be able to work out acceptable compromises. Both your lives have been affected by your illness but, if you view it as a joint problem and work as a partnership, it will make things a little easier.

Finally, a sense of humour helps. If you and your carer can laugh together about something that has happened, something that one of you has done, you are building a bond that will take you through the times when there may be much less to laugh at.

26 Improving your personal relationships

Illness often changes relationships. It puts a strain on both sides. You may be grieving for the past, for your lost job perhaps, for the things that you once could do, or for the changed image of yourself. However, your illness may have affected other people too. People close to you may also have a lot to grieve for. Carers may have had to take on the responsibility for housework or earning the money, and so have had to give up things they valued. They may be missing out on things they enjoyed previously on their own or with you. Their grief needs to be acknowledged too. You may feel that they are not caring enough; they may feel that you are asking too much. There may be a lot of resentment on both sides. All of this adds difficulties.

You may be feeling wounded that the friendships you had before you were ill do not seem to have survived. Often such friendships were based on doing things together—employment, sport, social activity—which are not possible for you now. Sometimes the relationship can be re-negotiated; sometimes it is no longer viable. It is important for your own well-being that you do your best to feel charitable about friends who have disappeared. Many people find illness in someone else an unwelcome reminder of their own potential vulnerability.

Emotions can get in the way of good relationships. If you are angry about ways in which you feel you have been misunderstood or mistreated, you may well be much more irritable than you used to be and bitter about life in general. This can make you a difficult person to be with. If you are wrapped up in your illness and concentrating a lot on your symptoms, you may well have less interest in the people around you. If you are very frustrated at what you now cannot do, you may be tempted to take it out on those close to you. Everything that we have said earlier about managing your emotions is especially important if you want to improve the way in which you get on with those around you.

Good communication really does help ease relationships, so we hope that you have found that what we wrote earlier gives you some idea of how you could improve things.

Some practical suggestions

Here are a few tips:

- Keep communications open. Avoid 'mind reading' (assuming that you know what the other person is thinking in a given situation). Your assumptions might be wrong.

- Check that the other person in the relationship knows the basic facts about your illness. Find simple ways of explaining to them how it affects you and what your limitations are.

- If something in the relationship is bothering you, choose a time when both of you are at your best to discuss the problem. Some people find that it helps to have a definite time once a week to talk over problems, with both sides having equal time to put their side of the picture.

- Do your best not to wait until you are in a rage and then explode with a grievance. You will be much more successful if you can explain your position calmly.

- Spend a little time imagining yourself in their place and thinking about things from their point of view. This can often let you see that they are not being as unreasonable as you first thought.

- Accept that some people are not going to understand what your illness is like for you. With some friends or relations, you may have to choose between going on seeing them, in spite of their lack of understanding, or cutting out that relationship for the time being. Do your best not to waste your energy getting worked up about the injustice of it.

- If something said to you makes you angry, give yourself time to calm down before you respond. The old saying about counting to 10 before you answer really is sensible.

- If relationships get very difficult and strained, it may be a good idea to seek professional help—family therapy or couple therapy for instance. Your doctor may be able to make suggestions as to how you could find such help.

- In general, try to aim for negotiation rather than confrontation.

Negotiation

It can often happen within a relationship that one person wants one thing whilst the other person wants something very different. It could be about something trivial such as which television programme to watch (though if you feel that your choices are always over-ruled it is not trivial), or it might be something much more serious. Either way, negotiation of the issue would be better than arguing about it. Ideally, it should end up with both people feeling that they have gained a reasonable part of what they want—a win–win outcome rather than one person winning and the other losing—in other words, collaboration.

It can be helpful if you consider your normal style of dealing with a confrontation. Do you:

- Go along with what the other person wants, perhaps because you feel they have more power, or for 'peace at any price'?
- Insist on getting what you believe are your rights?
- Avoid the confrontation, i.e. avoid the issue?
- Compromise in a way that perhaps means that neither side gets what they really want?

There may be circumstances in which any of these styles would be appropriate, but on a permanent basis they could lead to dissatisfaction.

Before you start the negotiation, it is very important that you are clear in your mind about the ideal result you would like, but also a fall-back position beyond which you would not go—'I could cope with such-and-such, but I wouldn't give way any more than that.'

There are several things that help:

- Be clear about what the issue is and do not get sidetracked into other ones.
- Find out what you agree about as well as what you disagree about.
- Be clear in your mind about what concessions you would be prepared to make.
- Stay calm. Getting angry or upset will hinder the negotiation.
- Stick to what you are discussing without criticizing the other person—say things like 'I'm unhappy when you do such-and-such' rather than 'You make me so unhappy.'
- Let the other person talk and listen carefully to what is said.

Both people could start the discussion by stating what they really want. Only after that should you suggest concessions or outline your fall-back position. To follow on from the example in the previous chapter:

Anna is a woman with rheumatoid arthritis who walks very slowly. Her husband Tom would like her to use a wheelchair when they are out shopping so that they could get things done faster, leaving more time to do the things he wants. Anna hates the idea of being seen in a wheelchair and being thought of as a cripple. So Tom wants her to use a wheelchair and Anna does not.

When Anna thinks about it carefully, she realizes that she might be prepared to use the wheelchair some of the time if it was different from their present one, which is a basic model that can only be pushed. Being in such a chair makes her feel more disabled. (People often think of someone being pushed in a different way from someone wheeling themselves.) She minds not being able to control it. Tom realizes that he does not need to use the wheelchair every time they are out.

The compromise they finally arrive at is that Tom will get a new light wheelchair that Anna can manoeuvre herself some of the time, but that they will only use it when he feels particularly pressed for time.

Further information

Manage your Mind, Gillian Butler and Tony Hope—Chapter 15
Getting to Yes: The Secret to Successful Negotiation, Roger Fisher and William Ury

Sexual relationships

If you have a partner, one of the areas that can cause difficulties is that of your sexual relationship. There may be many different reasons why you and your partner do not make love often or have given up on it altogether. It can be difficult to summon up much enthusiasm for sex if you are feeling unwell or in pain. You may even be afraid that the effort of making love could be dangerous to you. Similarly, the fear of hurting you, or even of causing you injury, can deter your partner. There may be aspects of your illness that make you feel less desirable. Some illnesses and the drugs used to treat them can reduce your enthusiasm for sex or affect performance or orgasm. You may have very limited mobility, which makes full intercourse difficult or painful. All of these things can have a bad effect on your sex life. Nevertheless, sex and loving are an important part of your relationship and something to be preserved if you can.

Being able to talk freely about sex is an important start. This may be difficult for both of you, particularly if it is something you have not done before. Persevere—it will get easier the more you do it. Both of you need to identify problems and discuss ways round them. Feel free to say what gives you pleasure and what does not, and encourage your partner to do the same. Talking in this way can be very exciting. If fear about the effort of making love is inhibiting either of you, check the facts about your illness and its effects. Ask your doctor or consultant about it. You may find that embarrassing, but they will not. Once you have done this, you could reassure your partner.

Change may be the key to greater success. If fatigue is getting in the way of your love life, consider different timing. Would the morning or afternoon suit you better than the evening? If pain is a problem, consider taking a painkiller at an appropriate time before love making is likely. Experiment with different positions that make things easier. It may be better to spend more time on foreplay and less time on penetrative sex. Forget about what you used to do and concentrate on what works for you now. One thing to consider is that giving pleasure can often be as satisfying as receiving it. Do believe that sex does not necessarily have to be just about passion; warmth and affection, closeness and cuddling can be just as important. Sex can be energizing as well as exhausting.

So far, we have been talking about an existing partnership. You may have the opportunity to start a new relationship, but the thought of potential difficulties with sex could deter you. When talking with this possible partner, it may be tempting to minimize the problems caused by your illness. This may be a short-term solution but could cause bigger problems later on. It might actually be quite a good test of whether that person was the right one for you to see how he or she reacts to knowing the full story.

Further reading

Living a Healthy Life with Chronic Conditions, Kate Lorig—Chapter 11

27 Your relationship with your doctors

If you have a long-term illness, the relationship you have with your doctor is important. It is worth thinking about what you can do to foster this key partnership. You both bring things to it—you bring your expertise and your experience of your illness and perhaps detailed medical information, your doctor brings expert medical knowledge, perspective, and judgement based on wider experience of illness in general. Even if this relationship is not too good at the moment, it may be possible to improve it. Clear, calm communication can be the key. It is in your own interest to be tactful, polite and quietly assertive rather than aggressive.

Being a patient with a long term-illness is quite different from the days when you only visited your doctor for something transient like a sore throat which could be addressed in one visit. You may be able to discuss this change with your doctor and together work out a new kind of partnership that fits the new circumstances.

- How often should you make an appointment and what would be a reason for making an appointment outside the normal schedule?
- What change in your symptoms should you report?
- What is the position about home visits if you are really too ill to get to the surgery?

If you have sorted all this out, it will prevent confusion or disappointment later.

Some people probably expect too much from their doctors. It can be helpful to distinguish between what you *need* (and are entitled to) from doctors and what you *want* from them. You *need* appropriate medical treatment (which is what they were trained to do), referral when appropriate to specialists and other sources of help, perhaps back-up when applying for benefits and, importantly, their objectivity and perspective when assessing information you bring to them. You may *want* emotional support (which they may not be able to provide). Concentrate on what you need from doctors and look elsewhere for what you want. Other sources for support and understanding could be your family or friends, local support groups for your particular illness or an online support group. If you cannot find it anywhere else, you could work on giving yourself emotional support.

Once you have sorted out in your mind what you need from doctors, it can also be helpful to look at things from their point of view. They have been trained to make a disease diagnosis and then to apply a specific treatment based on that diagnosis. This may make it difficult for them when there is no clear disease diagnosis or no effective treatment. Some doctors feel uneasy with chronic illnesses which they know they cannot cure. The relationship between you will probably be better if you can accept that there are limits to what doctors can offer. In particular, it will be helpful if you can acknowledge that, whilst they may not be able to offer a cure, they can help in other ways and that such help is very welcome.

Remember that doctors are people like you and that expecting them always to be on top form for you is unrealistic. For example, your doctor might have started the day by having a row with a partner, be feeling stressed by the pressures of bureaucracy, and now have a headache.

Being an 'expert patient'

An important element in the changed relationship between you and your doctor can come from you working towards being an 'expert patient' as we described in Chapter 3. Most doctors welcome this. Any partnership is based on mutual respect, so whilst you expect the doctor to respect your needs and expectations and to listen if you express some dissatisfaction, in turn it will help if you show that you respect their knowledge and experience.

Many people find it useful to search out information about their particular illness for themselves. However, when seeing doctors, it is probably best to select only the most relevant items and those that come from reputable sources. Do not turn up in the consulting room with a stack of print-outs from the Internet and necessarily expect doctors to welcome them. In Chapter 3 we gave advice on how to assess the likely accuracy and reliability of the medical information you find. Use this now. Think a little about *why* you want your doctor to see what you have found and what you expect them to do with the information. For instance, does it contain information about possible treatment for your illness that you have not yet been offered, or suggestions about reducing some of the symptoms? Acknowledge their wider medical knowledge, experience and perspective, perhaps by saying something like 'I would value your opinion on this'.

Unless you have one of the more common long-term illnesses, it is likely that you will come to know more about your illness than your doctor. General practitioners, as their name suggest, are generalists. They have to know about a broad range of medical conditions, but they cannot possibly be expert in all of them. Your doctor *may* find your condition particularly interesting and want to learn more about it, but could well consider that you would do better with an appropriate specialist. Even so, your doctor can still give you help with symptoms, and help you assess information you have found.

Listen carefully to what your doctor has to say about your illness. He or she may be telling you things you already know, but may be able to add something that you do not know.

The consultation

Doctors, particularly GPs, usually have much less time than they would like to spend with patients. A consultation with a GP is usually for only 7 or 8 minutes. If they over-run that time limit, it means that other patients will be kept waiting and probably get cross with the doctor, so if you can keep within the time limit it will be appreciated. How can you get all you want to say or discuss into such a short time? The key is good preparation. Take some time before the consultation to consider carefully what you want from it. Think about how you could express yourself clearly and succinctly. Take a check list with you and look at it before you leave, so that you do not come away realizing that you have missed out on something important.

- If you have a lot of questions you need to ask, list them in order of priority, as there may not be time to deal with all of them. You could give the doctor a copy of your check list (They can read more quickly than you can talk.) Ask yourself beforehand what kind of an answer you are looking for, as that can help you phrase the question accurately.

- If you do not understand the answers, ask for an explanation. This can be particularly important if the doctor uses medical terms you do not understand.

- If you are asked 'how are you?' it usually means 'how have you been?' Give clear details of how your symptoms have been since you last saw the doctor—have they stayed constant, improved or got worse—rather than making the doctor waste time digging the information from you. This would be a useful part of your preparation for the meeting.

- If pain is one of your problems, one way of rating it is on a scale of 1–10 (1 is minor pain; 10 is the worst you have experienced).

- If you have been experiencing side effects from a prescribed drug, describe them and find out if there are ways of minimizing them. You could ask if there is another drug with similar actions that might have fewer side effects.

- Do not leave something important to you to the last moment. Again, this is part of your preparation—ask yourself 'what is the one thing I want to tell the doctor or to find out?' and start with that.

- Your distress is part of the medical picture. You should feel free to say 'I am worried about such-and-such' or 'I find such-and-such a symptom particularly distressing'.

- It helps if you can demonstrate that you consider yourself a partner in your medical treatment. Show that you are ready to do what you can to help yourself. To give an example:

> John suffers from chronic back pain. At one of his check ups, the doctor finds that he is also suffering from hypertension (blood pressure raised higher than normal), and prescribes a drug to treat it. John agrees to take it, but asks if there is anything he can do for himself which would help. The doctor suggests that he give up smoking, lose some weight, increase the amount of exercise he takes and cut down on his drinking. At the next consultation John reports that he has taken the drug regularly. Though he has not managed to give up smoking completely, he has reduced it a great deal. He is now swimming twice a week and has lost three pounds. He has also reduced the amount he drinks. All this is welcomed by the doctor as it shows that they are working on John's problem together.

If you cannot get to the doctor, or have trouble choosing the right words when you do, try writing a brief letter explaining the problem and saying what you want. If you find it embarrassing to talk about a particular problem, you could put that in writing.

So far, we have talked about a consultation with a GP, but all that we have suggested can apply just as much to a consultation with a hospital specialist.

Specific requests to a doctor

You may want to ask for something more than routine care. You might think that it would be helpful if you had a particular test, perhaps an expensive one like an MRI scan. You might want to be referred to a specialist or to get a second opinion on your case. This can pose problems if not approached carefully. There are some things that you should think about or do before you make the request:

- Be clear in your mind *why* you want what you do. What do you hope to gain from it? Would the test you want lead to a different treatment or clear up doubts about your diagnosis? Do you believe that if you could only see the right specialist you could be offered a cure? If so, you are probably aiming for disappointment and your request is not likely to be well received. If, however, you think that a suitable specialist might be able to help you with a particular problem, then you are likely to do better. Make certain you have a good reason for what you are asking.

> Some years back, I got a referral to a leading general physician. I made it clear, both to my family doctor and then to the physician, that I was not looking for a cure for Chronic Fatigue Syndrome. As I was getting older, I realized that there might be other things happening because of increasing age. I wanted to be certain that not all my symptoms were due to CFS. Frankie

- Know the rules that apply to wherever you are living. Find out what limitations generally apply. For instance, in the UK, a doctor would need to produce a very special reason to refer a patient outside of his or her particular area. In America, there may be limitations of cost, perhaps depending on managed care incentives. Of course, if you are in a position to pay for a test or a consultation, you would have more choice.

- Be prepared to negotiate for what you want rather than just demanding it (see Chapter 26).

If you want to see a specialist or to get a second opinion, do your research first to find out as much as you can about which consultant would be likely to be of the greatest help. You could talk to other people who have the same illness as you do and ask them who they have found helpful. The manner of a particular doctor is one factor, but perhaps not the most important. What matters is that that doctor is really knowledgeable in his or her field. You could then say to your doctor something like 'If you agree, I would like to see Dr So-and-so'. If you do not have anyone particular in mind, ask your doctor's opinion.

Lack of continuity in which doctor you see

You may be lucky enough to be able to see the same doctor at each visit, whether a GP or a hospital specialist, but this unfortunately is becoming less usual. In some GP practices, it is difficult to make an appointment with just one doctor—you may have to accept an appointment with whoever is available. In these circumstances, it is even more important that you are very structured in your approach so that time is not wasted. It can be important to see that your symptoms and the things that you find difficult are recorded in your medical notes. If you are applying for financial benefits or practical help, you need to be certain that the appropriate information is available to whichever doctor happens to deal with this.

Remembering what you have been told

It is very easy to forget a great deal of what you have been told during a consultation. Research has shown that patients often retain only about a third of what they have been told by doctors. One way round this problem is to take someone with you. You may both forget some bits, but you are likely to cover more together. In hospital consultations, it is becoming more common to be offered a tape recording of the session. Do take up this offer if it is made. That way you can go over the consultation at your leisure and check that you have remembered and understood everything.

Medications

If you are prescribed a drug, it cannot do you any good if you do not take it! You may be reluctant to take any more drugs than is absolutely essential. Nevertheless, you will be presenting an inaccurate picture to the doctor if you accept a prescription and do not take the drug. Discuss your reluctance with the doctor and ask if there is an alternative to using the drug. You can find out more about any drug that has been prescribed by talking to your pharmacist, or by accessing one of the drug websites we listed in Chapter 3.

Make certain that your doctor is aware of any other drugs you are taking, even the ones that you may regard as 'natural' herbal remedies. Some of these can interact with prescribed medicines.

If your relationship with your doctor is unsatisfactory

There may be times when you feel that you are not getting what you want or need from your doctor. The first step is to think about what you would prefer to be getting and decide whether that is realistic. This has been discussed earlier in the chapter.

- Write down what you do get currently from your visits to your doctor, good and bad, and what you do not get. Describe for yourself what you would like to be getting, again staying realistic.

- Ask other people you know about what they get from their doctor. Compare your experience with theirs.

- Pay attention to your own style when you are with the doctor, to check whether how you are behaving might be part of the problem. Do you seem aggressive or do you demand a particular treatment rather than asking whether it would be appropriate? Do you waste time by being vague?

- Is the doctor's manner part of the problem? As long as the care given is effective, the manner is perhaps not so important.

- Perhaps the problem is in the organization of the practice rather than with the doctor—the receptionists may be rather unhelpful or you may have to wait a long time to get an appointment. You could discuss this with the practice manager.

If you are not getting what you would consider effective medical care, it is important to take steps to get what you need. This may mean explaining to your doctor just what you are not satisfied with—a very hard thing for most of us to do. Think yet again about whether your expectations are reasonable and then work out a diplomatic and polite way of expressing this. You may find it easier to do this in a letter to the doctor. If this does not work, then you may have to consider finding another doctor.

Changing your doctor

If, in spite of all your efforts, you decide that he or she is just not the right doctor for you and your condition, you could think about making a change. The simplest change is to switch to another doctor in the same practice, who may have a style that suits you more. If that is not possible, you could consider moving to another doctor's practice. Before you do this though, you should do as much research as possible. Most practices these days have brochures telling you about themselves, which can be some help. Probably the best source of information is word of mouth. Talk to as many patients of the possible doctors as you can to get a patients' eye view of them. You do not want to change one difficult doctor for another just as bad.

Medical systems in other countries

So far we have talked about the medical system and the National Health Service in the UK, which is obviously the one we know best. Though much of what we have said would apply to a relationship with a doctor in any country, there are differences that need to be looked at. If your health care is something you pay for directly or is covered by medical insurance, you may have more freedom to choose a doctor, though there may be some limitations set by your medical insurer. This may make it easier to change from a doctor who does not seem right for you, but there could be a temptation to go 'doctor shopping'. This can lead to you seeing doctor after doctor in the search for the perfect model, probably having more tests with each one you see.

Further information

The Patient's Internet Handbook, Robert Kiley and Elizabeth Graham—Chapter 12.

www.patients-association.com. This has a good section on dealing with doctors.

www.pocketdoctor.co.uk. This gives good suggestions about questions to ask your doctor in particular circumstances.

www.besttreatments.co.uk. This gives sound information about the best treatments for various medical conditions.

www.medic8.com. A good general information site. It includes a medical dictionary, which could be useful if you need to translate medical terms used by your doctor.

section 5
Managing practical problems

28 Improving your quality of life

In this chapter, we look at ways of making your life simpler or easier, so as to get the best from today. Improving the quality of your life today is a worthwhile aim. Making today better can also alleviate fears about tomorrow. Even if you believe that your health is not likely to improve, trying out some of the strategies we have suggested in this book may reduce some of your symptoms. Finding ways of overcoming some of the difficulties caused by your illness can improve the quality of your life. If you can feel that you are coping pretty well with what is happening now, you are more likely to feel more confident that you will cope with whatever tomorrow brings.

Making the most of a limited energy budget

If fatigue is one of your problems, you may well have to accept that the amount that you can do is limited, so it is worth thinking about whether everything you do is essential or pleasurable. Some people find it helpful to think in terms of budgeting their energy expenditure in the same way as they would budget a low income. You may have to make choices about whether you can afford something, whether it is in energy or money.

You could also think about whether you are 'spending' your energy efficiently. Using the same amount of energy to achieve a bit more is often possible if you think about it in a rather structured way. A good place to start is by considering your activities, mental as well as physical, under the headings of *What, Why, How* and *When* as we discussed in Chapter 8.

Changing the way in which you do things

If you are still doing things in the same way as you did before you became ill, you are likely to hit against obstacles and deny yourself possible pleasures or satisfactions. You may need to change your style quite a bit. One of the techniques that will help is to do a lot of forward planning, spreading out the task and pacing yourself carefully. Being too perfectionist will certainly get in the way.

> Clare has chronic fatigue syndrome (CFS/ME). She used to enjoy having friends round for a meal and had very high standards when she entertained. After a few bad experiences, trying to do things in the same old style, she realized that her friends did not expect her to do so much. She thought about very simple food that could be prepared well in advance—something like a casserole and a cold dessert—and got everything ready the previous day. To her delight she found that the social occasion was just as successful as before and yet it did not exhaust her.

With anything that you would like to do but that seems beyond you at the time being, think carefully about whether it would be possible if you tackled it in a rather different way.

Your home environment

We talked earlier about problem solving. You know better than anyone else about the problems caused by your illness that make your life at home more difficult. It is worth thinking this through, listing your problems, and then looking at ways of reducing them if not solving them. Getting expert help from someone such as an occupational therapist can be very useful.

Try standing back and looking at the place where you live. How could you make it more 'illness friendly'? De-cluttering your home can often make it much easier to clean and keep tidy.

If walking is a problem or if your balance is unsteady, then simplifying the layout of your rooms would probably be a good idea. Keep pathways through the rooms clear. Try to get into the habit of always putting things away after you have used them. Look carefully to check that there is nothing that you are likely to trip over.

Think about each room in turn:

- *The kitchen*—this is an important area. Could you rearrange things so that the items you use most frequently are easy to reach? Do you actually use or need everything there? Are there potential hazards that could be eliminated? Think about your specific difficulties and use problem-solving techniques to find solutions.

> When I took a hard look at my kitchen, I realized that I was still keeping a lot of plates and dishes from the time before I was ill when I used to give big buffet parties. Now that my style of entertaining had changed, they were mostly surplus to requirements. I gave a lot away to my family or to

charity shops and kept the things I really did use. This meant that I could reorganize my storage to make things much easier for myself. Frankie

- *The living room*—is there more in this room than you actually need? Would being a bit more minimalist make things easier? Is the chair you use most frequently suitable for your condition? Does it give good support to your back and head? Can you get out of it easily?

- *The bedroom*—getting the best quality sleep is important to you, so it is worth looking at your bed. If your mattress is more than 15 years old, it is probably time for a new one. If you still use blankets, you might find that changing to a duvet makes it easier to make the bed and eliminates a lot of dust. If you spend a lot of time resting there, could you make the room a more pleasant environment?

- *The bathroom*—there is a lot of equipment that can make bathing easier. Things like grab rails in appropriate places can make life a lot easier, both in getting in and out of the bath and in getting up from the toilet. Many people find that a walk-in shower with a folding seat can be very helpful.

Equipment

You may decide that there are various pieces of equipment that would make your life easier or allow you to do more with your available energy. There may be small or inexpensive things that would help—even a more efficient can-opener might be useful. In a book of this nature, aimed at people with a wide variety of different illnesses, it is not possible to be specific about the variety of aids and equipment available. Before you invest in anything expensive, it is well worth doing a lot of research. Resist the urge to rush into buying anything unless it is really cheap. See if there is a centre near you that displays such equipment, where you could look at what is available and try things out. Such centres often have a wide range of catalogues.

If you know other people with similar problems to yours, you could ask them what they have found useful. A home visit from an occupational therapist could be very helpful; he or she would be able to advise you on what equipment or alterations to your home would be appropriate. You may be one of the unlucky ones whose condition is likely to get worse. Thinking ahead of time about what equipment would then be necessary is a good idea.

If you enjoy gardening, but now experience difficulties with it, there is a wide range of specialist tools that could make things easier. You could try looking in your local garden centre to get ideas. You might consider reorganizing your garden to reduce effort. For instance, you might replace a lawn with paving, or have raised beds to eliminate bending. There are organizations in the UK and many other countries which can give you advice and information.

You do not have to think of equipment only in terms of practical problems. There may be something available that would make it possible to continue with a hobby.

Tom has MS. He now has problems with his hands. He has always enjoyed playing cards with his friends. When he began to have difficulty holding his cards, one of his friends looked in a catalogue and found larger sized cards and a rack to put them in. He also bought a gadget that shuffled the pack.

The subject of mobility aids can be a difficult one for some people. They may have very strong feeling about being seen with a walking stick and even stronger ones about using a wheelchair. Nevertheless, it is worth working through such feelings as the use of such aids can make a real difference to your quality of life.

I find it difficult and painful to walk more than a short distance. Some years ago, I realized that I was mostly seeing the world through glass—through either the windows of my house or my car. I bought myself an electric scooter, which enabled me to get back to walking my dog and being in the open air. I love it. Frankie

Employment

You may still be working, though perhaps with difficulty. What would be the best way of managing employment without putting too much strain on you? As we have said before, each person and each situation is different, so there are no hard and fast rules. However, we can offer some general, tried-and-tested suggestions.

First of all, it can be a great help if your immediate superior and your colleagues know about your illness and what it involves. However, this is not always desirable or possible. In some situations, it can have an adverse effect on career prospects to have it known that you have a health problem; some employers may be reluctant to take on a new employee with a record of ill health. You will have to be the best judge of this, but if you can be open about this, it will certainly make things easier.

If fatigue is one of your problems, you may have to accept that you will need to limit what you do in the evenings and at weekends and concentrate your energies on the working day. Pacing yourself while you are at work is very important. Try and give yourself pauses during which you switch off and relax.

Everything we have said about stress and stress management is particularly relevant in a working environment. It is worth giving a good deal of thought as to how you could reduce stress. Maybe you could go for a less demanding job; maybe you could get better at saying 'no' when unreasonable demands are made of you.

Communication and negotiation skills will certainly make your life easier. If the people around you do not understand about the limitations imposed on you by your illness, they may be resentful that you do not seem to be 'pulling your weight'. That would add to your problems.

29 Getting practical and financial assistance

Applying for practical help

Getting practical assistance with the things in your daily life which you find difficult, painful, fatiguing or even plain impossible can make managing your illness easier and improve your quality of life. Just how much help you need or would like will obviously depend on your particular illness and your individual circumstances. It is easy enough to talk about getting help, but in reality it can often be difficult. So where do you start looking?

The most obvious source of assistance is from partners, family, friends or neighbours. However, relying totally on such help could place too much of a burden on them. Thinking that they *ought* to help could be a source of deep misunderstanding and resentment. They may already be very much tied up in their own lives and their own problems and may not feel able to take on anything else. You need to think about their rights as well as your own. It helps if you can spread the load and not expect everything from just one person. Even if you are already getting such help, you may need more, so read on.

You may be able to get assistance from official sources, such as Social Services or through your family doctor's practice. Your doctor is often the gateway to such help, so do keep him or her informed about your needs. Mostly you have to be prepared to seek help actively. Just as you can take an active role in looking for information about your illness and its management from a wide variety of sources, you can do the same in searching in more than one place to find what help is available. If you have a long-term illness, you may have a right to certain kinds of practical assistance, which can include things such as housework and shopping, bathing and dressing, or help with transport. Obviously, what assistance you get can depend on your illness, your degree of disability and how overstretched local services are. Be prepared for filling out forms and perhaps talking about your financial position.

There are various organizations which will be able to give you information about what help you are entitled to and where to ask. We give some suggestions at the end of this section. It is worth spreading your net as wide as possible. There may be voluntary organizations locally, perhaps associated with a church, who can help in small ways.

It is important to be very clear in your own mind about what help you need and why, so that you can explain it in a way that other people, including officials, can understand. One thing that can get in the way of this can be a dislike of spelling out your problems and all the things you are no longer able to do. We do understand that this can be dispiriting. You may be only too aware of what these difficulties are, but putting them into words can be very depressing, particularly when talking to someone who does not seem to be sympathetic. You have to choose. If you want the help, you do need to talk about your problems, distasteful though this may be. Getting the right kind of help could make enough difference to your life to make it worth accepting the distress you feel when describing your difficulties.

If you can afford to buy help, then getting a cleaner to do some or all of your housework and shopping, or someone to take on the heavy jobs around the garden, can free you up to do more of the things that you enjoy or which give you satisfaction. Finding the right person is not always easy. A personal recommendation from a friend is useful, so ask around. It is a good idea to spell out exactly what you want done right from the start and establish a routine, so that on bad days you do not have to tell your helper what to do.

If you have always been independent, asking for help can be very difficult. Some people are very reluctant to ask for fear of having their request turned down. We talked more about this in Chapter 24. Just remember that having a request denied does not actually diminish you.

Sometimes it is the carer who needs help, but who may have to cope with not getting the necessary back-up from the person cared for (who may deny that any help is needed, perhaps because they resent hearing such things or are in denial about what they cannot do). There is no easy answer to this, except perhaps to cultivate a certain toughness of mind. Carers need to remind themselves that they have rights too.

Applying for financial benefits

Extra income can make illness a little easier and is worth seeking out. However, we are not going to talk about specific benefits here. Things change. Government legislation may alter existing benefits or bring in new ones. Out of date or inaccurate information would be of no use to you.

What we can talk about though are the general principles of applying for benefits.

To begin with, you need to know what benefits you might be entitled to and how to apply for them. Look at the list at the end of this section for possible sources of information.

It is important to be clear in your mind about the rules that apply to each benefit. What is it supposed to cover? For instance in the UK, the Attendance Allowance or the care element of Disability Living Allowance is given to provide money to pay for help in personal care for things such as washing, dressing and cooking meals, but not housework or shopping. When you are filling out the forms, include all the help that you need and why you need it, even if some of this is being covered by family or care workers. If you do not, you could miss out on a benefit you are entitled to. As an example, a woman we know whose husband did everything for her at the weekend was refused the level of benefit she deserved because she said that she only needed help 5 days a week. In reality, her actual need for help was the same weekdays or weekend. Some people when trying to think of what help they need find it helpful to imagine that they had a dedicated servant, and then think about what they would ask that servant to do.

Incapacity Benefit covers people who are unable to work because of illness. When filling out the application form, make certain that you put in all the facts that would back up your right to that particular benefit. Put in *all* the reasons why you are unable to work.

You may well need medical back-up for your claim. Make certain that your family doctor is aware of *all* your problems. It can be helpful to write out a clear list, to be included in your medical notes.

Some of the national support organizations for specific illnesses can give grants for things like equipment or holidays. It is always worth talking to them just in case.

Finding information and advice

In the UK, a good place to start is to look in the telephone Yellow Pages under headings such as Disability or Information Services. You could also talk to:

- Your local Citizens Advice Bureau
- The Social Services department of your local council
- The Benefits Helpline. You do not need to give your name when you ring this number
- The Claimants Union

- Help the Aged
- Age Concern
- Your local carers' group

You might also be able to get useful information from the local or national support group for your particular illness.

Further information

Living a Healthy Life with Chronic Conditions, Kate Lorig—Chapter 19. This gives details of accessing practical and financial help in the USA.

A Delicate Balance, Susan Milstrey Wells. Again, this gives advice about the American system

30 Thinking about the future

What about your future? Do you think about it? Some people with a long-term illness would rather not think about what might happen, but others prefer to make detailed plans for each eventuality. As in most things, a balance is probably best—somewhere between reasonable planning and excessive worry. Practical, constructive thought about how you could cope with future challenges could be very helpful, and may help you to be less fearful of what might happen. It could be sensible to discuss with your family doctor or consultant what the prognosis is in your particular condition. They may only be able to give you an informed, expert guess, but that might ease some of your fears.

If there are possible futures that you fear, you could make a list of them and then use problem solving (Chapter 16) to address each problem separately. In order to create possible solutions to each problem, you might need to do some research to find out what resources would be available to you, or what practical help might be available locally. You could find out about what equipment or what alterations to your home might be of benefit and whether there are any grants or financial help towards them. If restricted mobility could be a problem, then you could think about ways of dealing with that, such as adaptations to your car, or getting a wheelchair or an electric scooter. If it is possible that you might need some form of sheltered housing, then you could find out what is available locally and get your name on a waiting list. This does not commit you to anything.

You might need to think about your family's reaction to any possible worsening in your condition. This could be something that they have already considered, but have hesitated to mention for fear of upsetting you, or they may prefer to deny the possibility. Talking it over in an unemotional way might be constructive.

Getting older

One thing that is certain is that, ill or not, we all get older year by year, and ageing often brings other problems that will add to your existing illness. The older you get, the more likely it is that you will experience other medical conditions. So planning ahead of time for the reduction in ability that ageing can bring is very sensible. It could be helpful to think about what changes would need to be made to allow you to stay as independent as possible for as long as possible.

You could think about adaptations to your house or to your garden to make them both less labour intensive. You might find it helpful to do some research about gadgets and equipment that could make caring for yourself easier.

However, you might decide that your present house and your present garden would not be suitable as you get older. Planning well ahead of time could make a move easier. Keeping an eye on the local housing market could give you an idea of what more suitable housing might be available. If you have lived in your present home for some years, you will probably have accumulated a lot of clutter (most of us do), so 'de-cluttering' at your leisure could make a move much less stressful.

Some families adapt their houses to provide a 'granny flat' for a parent. This can have both advantages and disadvantages for both sides, and is not something to be decided on in a hurry.

Would you want to stay in the same area you live in now when you, or a partner, reach retirement age? Many people have dreams of moving to the country or to the sea. This could be feasible, but it is always worth thinking this through in depth and doing as much research as you can before you make a move. If you did move, would you miss the friends you have now or be able to make new ones? What would the medical services be like in the new location? Would it be easy to find suitable, affordable housing there? (Housing costs vary very much from area to area.) Maybe you could arrange to have a local newspaper delivered for a while so that you could find out more about the facilities and house prices.

Whether you decide to move away from your present area, or just to move into something more suitable for increasing age, it is worth doing it while you still feel able to make a move without too much difficulty.

I am making plans to move to a smaller house, with a much smaller garden. I want to make the move while I still have the capacity to do so. Meanwhile, I am researching all the things that would make the next house as disabled/ elderly friendly as possible. Even small things could help, such as levers on all ~)s instead of knobs, and electric sockets at waist height where appropriate.

I want to stay within the area covered by my very good doctor, but move closer to a bus service, so that I would not be dependent on being able to drive. Frankie

Perhaps in time, you might need more assistance than you could get in your own home. As we suggested earlier, could you look at sheltered housing or warden-assisted apartments?

It is certainly a good idea to keep yourself interested and mentally active as you get older. There is evidence that keeping our brains exercised as we get older is very important. Keep up with your hobbies if you can, or find new ones. Do your best not to lose touch with friends and perhaps find ways to make new ones. You might choose to join a lunch club, or take part in other such activities. We know of many older people who still go on learning—going to classes or taking courses in their own homes.

Exercise is important too. You will want to stay as mobile as possible, and appropriate exercise will help with this. Of course it may need to be tailored to your particular condition, but gentle swimming and walking will do you a lot of good. You may find classes in your area that specialize in helping older people.

Thinking about dying and death

We hope we are not thought to be morbid in introducing this topic. Though everybody knows intellectually that they will die sometime, we may at an emotional level think of ourselves as immortal, not accepting death as the inevitable last stage of a journey through life. If you are living with a long-term illness, you may become more aware of your own mortality than some other people. There is no 'right' way or 'wrong' way of thinking about dying. You can choose not to think about it at all if that is your way of dealing with it. Probably you will deal with death in much the same way as you dealt with life.

Some people would feel more comfortable if they knew that their affairs were in order and that they were not leaving a lot for their families to sort out after their death. If you have not yet made a will, it is really sensible to do something about it now. If you die intestate (not having made a will), it can cause enormous problems for those you leave behind. If you have very little to leave, you can make a simple will using a special form obtainable at stationers, or you can download a will form from the Internet. However, it is probably better to use the services of a lawyer if you can afford it.

Many people fear dying rather than death itself. They are afraid that process will be very unpleasant or painful. They hope for a 'good d but picture something very different. One definition of a good death is 'with dignity, among friends and without pain'. If you can bring yourself to think about such a subject, how would you like your end to come? No one can control the future totally, but you can make some of your wishes known in advance.

You may hope that doctors will do everything in their power to prolong your life as long as possible, or you might prefer them to concentrate on keeping you as comfortable as they can, without using extreme measures to give you a few more days or weeks. You could talk this over with your family, so that they know your wishes. Some people choose to set down in writing a 'living will'—a detailed instruction about what they want or do not want. It could be helpful if you also discuss this with your doctor, so that your wishes are included in your health notes.

Do realize that the concept of palliative care has spread beyond hospices. Most hospitals have a palliative care team, who can help a patient to be more comfortable. Pain control is becoming increasingly sophisticated, so you do not need to fear dying in extreme pain. There are moves now to extend palliative care to people in their own homes.

Some people at some point enjoy planning their own funerals; others would much rather not think of it at all. Whichever way suits you is right for you. Maybe you could check with your close family and find out what they would prefer.

You could think about what things you would prefer not to leave undone—the thing you meant to say to somebody, the reconciliation with someone you have quarrelled with. It is often said that it is easier to face the end of life if there are few regrets about unfinished business.

Summary

The theme of this book has been the idea that self-management, combined with medical help, is the best way for someone with a long-term illness to improve their general well-being and to obtain a better quality of life. Self-management can be much more than just working on reducing symptoms, though that is obviously important. You can look at all aspects of your life—physical, emotional, social and practical. You know yourself and your circumstances better than anyone else can. You know where improvements can be made.

If you have reached this point in the book, you will have read about various aspects of long-term illness in general, including the biopsychosocial model and the concept of self-management:

- Ideas about illness and ways of managing it
- Ways of seeking out information and becoming an 'expert patient'
- Ways of managing physical problems
- Emotional aspects of illness
- The importance of relationships and how to improve them
- Some practical and social issues.

All of these are tools and equipment that you could use to help you along the journey which is your illness. You are unique, so probably only some of these tools may be useful to you. You perhaps skipped the bits that did not interest you, which is perfectly OK, though you may find at a later stage that you want to go back to some of them.

It does not have to stop here though. You can go on adding to your tool box and working on improvements. These may be small, but together they could add up to something significant. As you journey on, there are bound to be changes, whether in the progress of your illness or in things that happen just because you are getting older. It can be tempting to think something like 'Well I've sorted out my self-help programme. I don't need to think about that again', but staying flexible about what you do to help yourself is important. Be prepared to look at new ideas.

One thing to consider is the 'ripple' effect. Anything you can do for yourself, or be helped to do, that improves one aspect of your life almost always affects other aspects. If you can improve one or more of your symptoms, then that will usually improve your emotional state. Equally, an improvement in your emotional state can have a good effect on your physical state. Getting better at communicating with those around you reduces stress, and that is likely to be good for your body, as well as making you feel better emotionally. Getting help with the things you find difficult or getting financial assistance can make a real difference to your quality of life.

Something you can look forward to is a slow improvement in the way that doctors and health professionals work with long-term illness. There are very definite moves in that direction. It is very likely that doctors will come to see that a partnership with their long-term patients is what is needed, and that they may look to such patients to teach them how to improve their services. Just as an example, on March 19, 2005, the *British Medical Journal* (which is widely read and has a lot of influence) published a theme edition on chronic illness, covering just these points. One thing that was said was 'What can we learn from our patients about the best way of helping them?' Of course, getting better care from your doctors would be very nice, but the whole message of this book has been that what you do to help yourself is even more important.

There are many ideas in this book about ways in which you might help yourself, but just reading about them is not enough. Only you can decide which ones might be appropriate to you, and only you can make the changes to incorporate those ones into your everyday life. Our hope is that you will try at least some of them and find that they help. You have our very best wishes for your journey.

F.C. and M.S.

Appendix 1   The DISCERN instrument

The DISCERN instrument was designed to help patients assess the quality of written information about treatment choices. It can be applied to printed material or to something found online. It really can help you be more 'discerning' about something that may, at first sight, appear to be quite sound and to spot its weaknesses. If you have access to a computer, it is worth calling up the website www.discern.org.uk/discern_instrument. If you click onto 'rating this question', you will be given even more help in answering each question.

We are very grateful to have been given permission to reproduce it for you in this book.

General instructions

The questions

DISCERN consists of 15 key questions plus an overall quality rating. Each of the 15 questions represents a separate **quality criterion**—an essential feature or standard that is an important part of good quality information on treatment choices.

The questions in DISCERN are organized in three sections as follows:

Questions 1–8 address the reliability of the publication and should help you consider whether it can be trusted as a source of information about treatment choices

Questions 9–15 focus on specific details of the information about treatment choices. Please note:

- Apart from question 14, the questions are concerned with the treatment choice or choices described **in the publication** and not with all treatment choices
- Questions 1–11 are concerned with the 'active' treatments described in the publication and can include self-care. 'No treatment' options are dealt with separately in Question 12

Question 16 is the overall quality rating at the end of the instrument. Your answer to this question should be based on your judgement of the quality of the publication as a source of information about treatment choices after rating each of the preceding 15 questions. However, you should only rate a publication as good quality if it rated well on the majority of questions.

Occasionally, a question is not appropriate for a publication. For example, the question about no treatment options would not be appropriate for a publication about labour and birth. You should use your judgement to exclude a question that is not relevant. However, DISCERN has been developed as an **appraisal process** and should be used in its entirety. You must not use individual questions of sets of questions separately.

You will find it easiest to read the publication fully before answering the DISCERN questions

The rating scale

Each question is rated on a 5-point scale ranging from No to Yes. The rating scale has been designed to help you decide whether the quality criterion in question is present or has been 'fulfilled' by the publication. General guidelines are as follows:

- **5** should be given if your answer to the question is a definite 'yes'—the quality criterion has been completely fulfilled
- **Partially (2–4)** should be given if you feel the publication being considered meets the criterion **to some extent**. How high or low you rate 'partially' will depend on your judgement of the extent of these shortcomings
- **1** should be given if the answer to the question is a definite 'no'—the quality criterion has not been fulfilled at all

Hints

A number of hints are given after each question. These are designed to provide you with things to look for or consider when deciding your response to a question. The hints should act as a guide rather than as hard and fast rules, and your own judgement will also be important. The rating process is clear cut for most questions, although more subjective decisions may occasionally be needed. The hints should help you to use your own judgement effectively in all cases. More specific instructions are given for questions 2, 4 and 5.

Additional guidance

Additional guidance for rating each question is provided with the instrument. Click on 'Rating this question' (*if you are looking at it on the website*) if you are having difficulties and would like to understand the issues underlying a question more fully. We have included an example of a Yes, Partially and No rating wherever possible. The examples have been developed from written consumer health information and are purely fictitious. Any resemblance to a real publication is purely coincidental. In some cases, it has not been possible to provide concise examples of the full range of ratings, but you should be able to work out an appropriate response from the instructions and the examples given.

Remember: throughout the DISCERN instrument and website:

- **treatment** includes self-care
- **treatment choices** are possible treatment options including no treatment
- **information** refers to information about treatment choices only
- a **publication** is any written item that provides information about treatment choices specifically for health consumers, and can include printed and online materials.

The DISCERN instrument

SECTION 1. Is the publication reliable?

1. Are the aims clear?

Rating this question

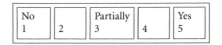

HINT Look for a clear indication at the beginning of the publication of:

- What it is about
- What it is meant to cover (and what topics are meant to be excluded)
- Who might find it useful
- If the answer to Question 1 is 'No', go directly to question 3

2. Does it achieve its aims?

Rating this question

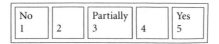

HINT Consider whether the publication provides the information it aimed for as outlined in Question 1

3. Is it relevant?

Rating this question

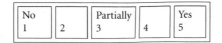

HINT

- The publication addresses the question that readers might like to ask
- Recommendations and suggestions concerning treatment are realistic and appropriate

4. Is it clear what sources of information were used to compile the publication (other than the author or producer)?

Rating this question

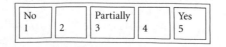

HINT

- Check whether the main claims or statements made about treatment choices are accompanied by a reference to the sources used as evidence, e.g. a research study or expert opinion.
- Look for a means of checking the sources used such as a bibliography/reference list or the addresses of the experts or the organizations quoted or external links to the online sources.

Rating note: in order to score a full '5', the publication should fulfil both hints. Lists of **additional** sources of support and information (Question 7) are not necessarily sources of **evidence** for the current publication.

5. Is it clear when the information used or reported in the publication was produced?

Rating this question

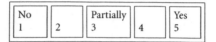

No 1	2	Partially 3	4	Yes 5

HINT Look for:

- dates of the main sources of information used to compile the publication
- date of any revisions of the publication (but not dates of reprinting in the case of print publications)
- date of publication (copyright date)

6. Is it balanced and unbiased?

Rating this question

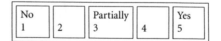

No 1	2	Partially 3	4	Yes 5

HINT Look for:

- a clear indication of whether the publication is written from a personal or objective point of view
- evidence that a **range** of sources of information was used to compile the publication, e.g. more than one research study or expert
- evidence of an external assessment of the publication

Be wary if:

- the publication focuses on the advantages or disadvantages of one particular treatment choice without reference to other possible choices
- the publication relies primarily on evidence from single cases (which may not be typical of people with this condition or of responses to a particular treatment)
- the evidence is presented in a sensational, emotive or alarmist way.

7. Does it provide details of additional sources of support and information?

Rating this question

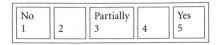

HINT Look for suggestions for further reading or for details of other organizations providing advice and information about the condition and treatment choices.

8. Does it refer to areas of uncertainty?

Rating this question

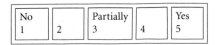

HINT

- Look for discussion of the gaps in knowledge or differences in expert opinion concerning treatment choices.
- Be wary if the publication implies that a treatment choice affects everyone in the same way, e.g. 100% success rate with a particular treatment.

SECTION 2. How good is the quality of information on treatment choices?

N.B. The questions apply to the treatment or treatments described **in the publication.** Self-care is considered a form of treatment throughout this section.

9. Does it describe how each treatment works?

Rating this question

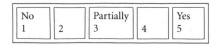

Hint Look for a description of how a treatment acts on the body to achieve its effect.

10. Does is describe the benefits of each treatment?

Rating this question

No 1	2	Partially 3	4	Yes 5

HINT Benefits can include controlling or getting rid of symptoms, preventing recurrence of the condition and eliminating the condition, both short term and long term.

11. Does it describe the risks of each treatment?

Rating this question

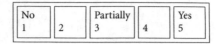

HINT Risks can include side effects, complications and adverse reactions to treatment, both short term and long term.

12. Does it describe what would happen if no treatment is used?

Rating this question

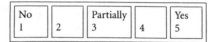

HINT Look for a description of the risks and benefits of postponing treatment, of watchful waiting (i.e. monitoring how the condition progresses without treatment) or of permanently forgoing treatment.

13. Does it describe how the treatment choices affect overall quality of life?

Rating this question

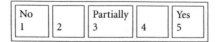

HINT Look for:

- Description of the effects of the treatment choices on day-to-day activity
- Description of the effects of the treatment choices on relationships with family, friends and carers.

14. Is it clear that there may be more than one possible treatment choice?

Rating this question

No 1	2	Partially 3	4	Yes 5

HINT Look for:

- A description of who is most likely to benefit from each treatment choice mentioned, and under what circumstances
- Suggestions of alternatives to consider or investigate further (including choices not fully described in the publication) before deciding whether to select or reject a particular treatment choice.

15. Does it provide support for shared decision making?

Rating this question

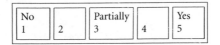

| No 1 | | 2 | | Partially 3 | | 4 | | Yes 5 |

HINT Look for suggestions of things to discuss with family, friends, doctors or other health professionals concerning treatment choices.

SECTION 3. Overall rating of the publication

16. Based on the answers to all of the above questions, rate the overall quality of the publication as a source of information about treatment choices

Rating this question

Low		Moderate		High
Serious or extensive shortcomings		Potentially important but not serious shortcomings		Minimal shortcomings
1	2	3	4	5

Copyright British Library and the University of Oxford

Appendix 2 Further information

Here are the full details of all the books, websites, etc. that you will have noticed as 'Further information' at the end of sections throughout the book. We have also listed other books, audio cassettes and CDs, and websites which we think will be of use to you and which expand what we have been able to fit into just one book.

You may well be able to borrow some of the books from a library. Most of the titles we suggest are available from Amazon.

Long-term illness and its management

Living a Healthy Life with Chronic Conditions. Kate Lorig, Halstead Holman, David Sobel, Diana Laurent, Virginia Gonzalez and Marian Minor. Bull Publishing Company, 2003—an American book on self-management. ISBN 0923521534.

A Delicate Balance. Susan Milstrey Wells. Insight Books, 1998—an American book giving a view of illness within the US health care system. ISBN 0306457899.

Coping with Long-term Illness. Barbara Baker. Sheldon Press, 2001—another slant on long-term illness. ISBN 0859698440.

Living Creatively with Chronic Illness. Eugenie G. Wheeler and Joyce Dace-Lombard. Pathfinder Publishing, 1989—an inspirational book on developing the skills to transcend loss, pain and frustration. ISBN 0934793174.

Getting to Yes: The Secret to Successful Negotiation. Roger Fisher and William Ury. Random House Business Books, 2003—a good book if you want to learn more about negotiation and communication styles. ISBN 1844131467.

Oxford Concise Medical Dictionary. Oxford University Press—helpful if you do not understand some of the medical terms you hear or read. ISBN 119280085X.

CancerBACUP—3 Bath Place, Rivington Street, London EC2A 3DR, www.cancerbacup. org.uk—this organization produces a series of very good, free booklets dealing with all aspects of cancer. '5 Steps to Living Everyday—Coping with cancer-related fatigue' is particularly good and can be applied to lots of other conditions.

Looking after yourself

The Which? Guide to Complementary Therapy. Barbara Rowlands. Which? Books, 1997—a good guide to complementary and alternative therapies, with sensible suggestions about choosing a therapist. ISBN 085202634X.

Back in Ten Minutes. Dr May Rintoul and Bernard West. Penguin, 1995—a very practical book about ways of avoiding back problems. It contains really clear illustrations of suggested exercises. ISBN 0140234829.

A Survival Guide to Later Life. Marion Shoard. Constable and Robison, 2004—helpful if you are thinking about the added problems of increasing age. ISBN 1841193720.

A Complete Guide to Massage. Susan Mumford. Hamlyn, 2000—will give you ideas about massage you can do yourself or train someone else to do. ISBN 0600599922.

Managing More with Less. Joanna Howard. Butterworth Heinemann, 1997—though this book is aimed at people at work, most of what it says can be applied to normal life. ISBN 075063698X.

Managing pain

Pain: The Science of Suffering. Patrick Wall. Weidenfeld and Nicolson, 1999—an interesting and compassionate book about pain. ISBN 0297842552.

Coping Successfully with Pain. Nevil Shone. Sheldon Press, 1995—techniques for self-help with chronic pain. ISBN 0859698505.

Bandolier's Little Book of Pain. Moore, Edwards, Barden and McQay, Oxford University Press, 2003—evidence-based details of the best ways of treating a wide range of pain conditions. ISBN 0192632477.

Being a carer

The Selfish Pig's Guide to Caring. Hugh Marriott. Polperro Heritage Press, 2003—a practical and realistic book about the problems of being a carer, written by someone who is a carer himself. ISBN 0954423313.

Caring for Someone at a Distance. Julie Spencer-Cingoz. Age Concern, 1998—a helpful book about caring for someone who does not live with you. ISBN 0863422280.

Meditation

Full Catastrophe Living. Jon Kabat-Zinn, Piatkus 1990—an introduction to the techniques of mindfulness meditation and its use in dealing with stress and pain. ISBN 0749915854.

Science of Being and Art of Living—Transcendental Meditation. Marharisshi Mahesh Yogi. Plume Books, 2001, ISBN 0452282667.

Change Your Mind: Guide to Buddhist Meditation. Pamananda. Windhorse Publications, 1996. ISBN 0904766810.

How Does Meditation Heal—A Practical Guide to Healing Your Mind and Body. Eric Harrison, 2000—a short but useful book. ISBN 0749921099.

Using the Internet

The Patient's Internet Handbook. Robert Kiley and Elizabeth Graham. The Royal Society of Medicine Press, 1998—an invaluable book if you want to look for medical information on the Internet. ISBN 1853154989.

Help with your emotions

Manage Your Mind. Gillian Butler and Tony Hope, Oxford University Press, 1995—one of the best self-help books, covering a wide range of subjects. It is written in a very clear way and is full of common sense. It has good chapters on dealing with worry and anxiety, problem solving, relationships and communications. ISBN 0192623834.

Overcoming Anxiety. Helen Kennerly. Constable and Robinson, 1998—self-help techniques for dealing with anxiety. ISBN 1854874225.

Panic Attacks. Christine Inghams. Thorsons, 1993—self-help techniques for dealing with panic. ISBN 0007106904.

Overcoming Depression. Paul Gilbert. Constable and Robinson, 1997—self-help techniques for dealing with depression. ISBN 1841191256.

Overcoming Low Self-esteem. Melanie Fennell. Constable and Robinson, 1999—one of the best books on the subject. ISBN 1854877259

Mind Over Mood. Dennis Greenberger and Christine Padesky. Guilford Press, 1995—one of the best books about cognitive behaviour therapy self-help techniques for dealing with anxiety, panic and depression. ISBN 0898621283.

The Which? Guide to Counselling and Therapy. Mike Brookes and Shamil Wanigaratne. Which? Books, 2003—a very helpful book which explains what is involved in counselling and different psychotherapies, as well as giving sensible advice on choosing a therapist. ISBN 0852029233.

Useful websites

www.quackwatch.com provides practical advice on how to identify rogue sites on the Internet dealing with complementary and alternative therapies.

www.continence-foundation.org.uk gives very helpful information and advice about bladder and bowel problems. You can use it to find a local continence clinic in the UK. There are similar organizations in Canada and Australia.

www.carers.org The Princess Royal Trust for Carers offers useful information and support for all unpaid carers throughout the UK.

www.changingfaces.org.uk offers advice and support to people with facial or bodily disfigurement.

Drug information

www.bnf.org is the website of the *British National Formulary*. You may have seen the book on your doctor's desk.

www.intelihealth.com is the website for the *US Pharmacopoeia*.

Good sources of information about illnesses and treatments

www.nhsdirect.nhs.uk is the website for the information service NHS Direct.

www.bandolier.org.uk is an evidence-based website giving sound information about treatment.

www.mayoclinic.com is an American site giving sound and reliable information about a variety of medical conditions.

www.healthtalk.com is an American site that aims to give the latest information about treatments and disease management.

www.medic8.com is an interesting site on a variety of medical conditions. It contains a medical dictionary.

Pain

www.iasp-pain.org is the website for the International Association for the Study of Pain. It gives helpful information on a range of pain issues, as well as suggesting some useful links.

www.inputpainunit.net is the website for the Guy's and St Thomas' Hospital main management unit. It has interesting information about self-management techniques, a good reading list and some useful links to other sites.

How to get the best results from your doctor

www.pocketdoctor.co.uk gives examples of questions to ask your doctor in a variety of circumstances.

www.patients-association.com has a good section on dealing with doctors.

www.besttreatments.co.uk gives sound information about the best treatments for various medical conditions.

Audio-cassettes and CDs

Talking Life at www.talkinglife.co.uk, PO Box 1, Wirrall CH47 7DD, UK, 01516321206— is a good source of tapes and CDs on a variety of subjects. We can thoroughly recommend their Relaxation Kit, Coping with Pain, Coping with Anxiety, and Coping with Depression. It could be worth getting their catalogue.

Another good relaxation tape is available from: Oxford Cognitive Therapy Centre, Warneford Hospital, Oxford OX3 6JX, UK, 01865223986.

A good CD dealing with managing chronic pain is: Living with chronic pain by Neil Berry, 2001, available from Pain CD, PO Box 84, Blackburn, BB2 7GH, UK. It ends with a good track on relaxation.

Appendix 3 Papers from medical journals

Baker, M.G. and Graham, L. (2004) The journey: Parkinson's disease. *British Medical Journal* 329, 611–614.

Bodenheimer, T., Lorig, K., Holman, H. and Grumbach, K. (2002) Patient self-management of chronic disease in primary care. *Journal of the American Medical Association* 288, 2469–2475.

Holman, H. and Lorig, K. (2004) Patient self-management: a key to effectiveness and efficiency in care of chronic disease. *Public Health Reports* 119, 239–243.

Lorig, K. (2002) Partnerships between expert patients and physicians. *Lancet* 359, 814–815.

McCracken, L.M., Carson, J.W., Eccleston, C. and Keefe, F.J. (2004) Acceptance and change in the context of chronic pain. *Pain* 109, 4–7.

Newman, S., Steed, L. and Mulligan, K. (2004) Self-management interventions for chronic illness. *Lancet* 364, 1523–1537.

Von Korff, M., Gruman, J., Schaefer, J., Curry, S.J. and Wagner, E.H. (1997) Collaborative management of chronic illness. *Annals of Internal Medicine* 127, 1097–1102.

Von Korff, M., Glasgow, R.E. and Sharpe, M. (2002) Organising care for chronic illness. *British Medical Journal* 325, 92–94.

Warsi, A., Wang, P.S., LaValley, M.P., Avorn, J. and Solomon, D.H. (2004) Self-management education programs in chronic disease: a systematic review and methodological critique of the literature. *Archives of Internal Medicine* 164, 1641–1649.

Wright, E.B., Holcombe, C. and Salmon, P. (2004) Doctors' communication of trust, care, and respect in breast cancer: qualitative study. *British Medical Journal* 328, 864.

Ziebland, S., Chapple, A., Dumelow, C., Evans, J., Prinjha, S. and Rozmovits, L. (2004) How the internet affects patients' experience of cancer: a qualitative study. *British Medical Journal* 328, 564.

index